Live Healthy

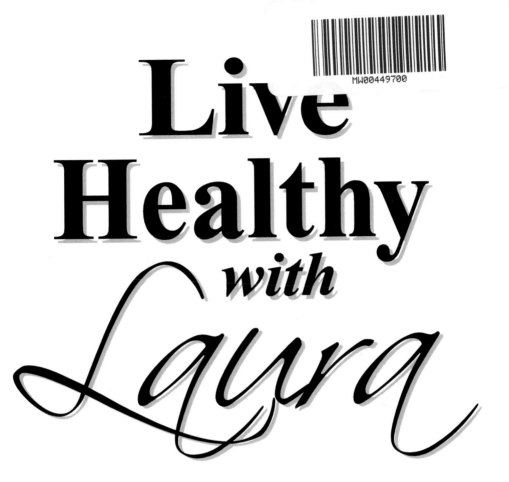

with

Laura

Live Healthy
with
Laura

*Stop Dieting and Start Living with my
10 Easy to Follow Lifestyle Principles,
30 of my Favorite Recipes and More!*

LAURA HEFLIN

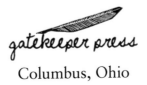

gatekeeper press

Columbus, Ohio

Live Healthy with Laura: Stop Dieting and Start Living with my 10 Easy to Follow Lifestyle Principles, 30 of my Favorite Recipes and More!

Published by Gatekeeper Press
2167 Stringtown Rd, Suite 109
Columbus, OH 43123-2989
www.GatekeeperPress.com

ISBN (paperback): 9781662901140
eISBN: 9781662901157

Library of Congress Control Number: 2020940760

To my husband and kids.
I love you more than words can say.
Thank you for all of your love and support
and for giving me even more of a
reason to live a healthy life!

Disclaimer:

This book is intended only as an informative guide. In no way is this book intended to replace, countermand, or conflict with the advice given to you by your own physicians and dieticians or any other medical professional. The ultimate decisions concerning care should be made between you and your doctor. I strongly recommend you follow his or her advice. Information in this book is general and offered with no guarantees on the part of the authors or publisher. The authors and publisher disclaim all liability in connection with the use of this book. Mention of specific companies, organizations, products, or authorities in this book does not imply endorsement by the author or publisher, nor does the mention of specific companies, organizations, products, or authorities imply that they endorse this book.

Contents

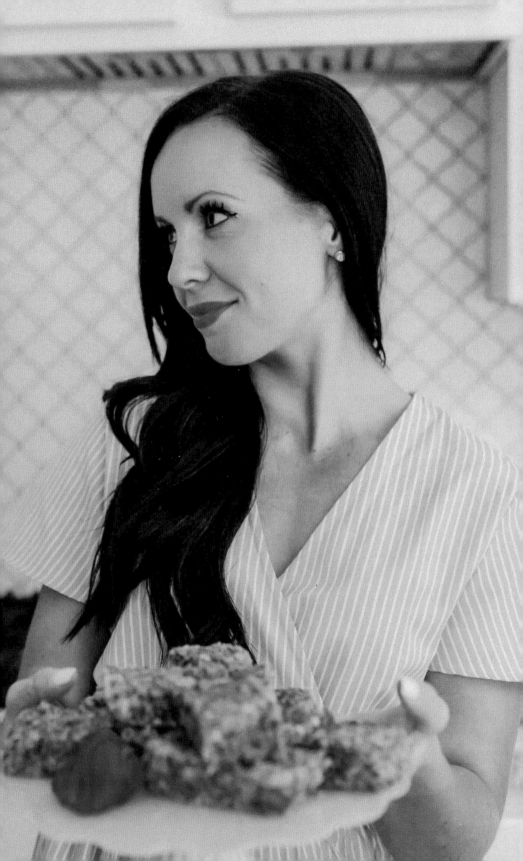

Introduction

Food brings me such joy. When I get into my kitchen, I see my blank counter space as a canvas and the various ingredients around my kitchen as my palate. I follow my heart and my stomach and I get in the kitchen and bring a new creation to life every chance I get. To me, the kitchen is my happy place and my escape from the busy world we live in. I see food as a means to nourish our bodies and a way to bring more joy into our lives. I see food as a never-ending sea of tastes and textures. The sky is really the limit! I think it's important to remember that what we put in our bodies is so incredibly powerful! It can heal us or it can harm us. I wrote this book to take a stand against the stigma of healthy eating. I want to express to the world that healthy eating can and should taste delicious and leave you feeling amazing and light on your feet. It is *not* about calories in, calories out. It is about what our food can do for our body! **I believe that food should be as good for you as it tastes!** That's my motto!

Oh, how my mindset has changed since a decade ago when food, to me, was a way of just getting by and manipulating my body to simply weigh less. The fewer calories a meal or snack was, the better. Yes, that is, sadly, how I truly thought. I didn't stop to think about *what* I actually was fueling my body with. I just cared that I was sticking to a certain calorie limit. Naturally, of course, a lot of whole foods are low in calories, so I ended up eating mostly well, but still, it wasn't with a healthy mindset. I quickly lost the weight that I had gained in the early years of marriage, plus a few extra pounds, but I was depressed and miserable. My body and brain were starved for nutrition! My hormones were all over the place and I began to resent food.

If I wanted something "indulgent," I would distract myself and deprive myself of it. I thought if I did that, I was taking control of my cravings. I thought I was "being good." It was a very depressing time in my life, but it led me to where I am today.

Today I am grateful for those hard times and more in love with food than ever. I like to now refer to myself as a "foodie." I am no longer afraid of any particular food but instead I eat freely—and I am the healthiest I have ever been! I want to feel my best, so I choose the best ingredients possible to leave my taste buds content and my body happy. Truly, though, I eat whatever my heart desires, in moderation, and I want to teach you to do the same! In this book, I want to introduce you to the "Live Healthy With Laura" way of life. I want to teach you that food can and should taste delectable and you should never run from it. This lifestyle gives you room to eat what you love in moderation and without a single moment of guilt! In this book, you will learn how to develop a beautiful relationship with food and how to eat what you crave while staying mindful of your health at the same time. *Nothing* is off-limits! Life is short and though I want you to be healthy, I also want you to enjoy each and every day—and I want you to live free!

10 Lifestyle Principles

Principle One: *Don't Start Something Today You Can't Do the Rest of Your Life*

It is no secret that we live in such an extremist culture, with an "all or nothing" mentality. You either diet and eat like a rabbit all day or you binge on the entire carton of ice cream. There is no in-between. Sadly, I think our culture has forgotten the concept of *balance*. We have forgotten how to enjoy food and how to listen to our body when it is telling us what it needs. We have lost sight of the fact that healthy food doesn't have to be bland and void of flavor or premade for us and delivered to our front door. We have forgotten what it's like to be in the kitchen, creating food from scratch, because processed fast foods and premade meals are just so easy to access these days.

Every single day I can scroll through social media and come across another new diet headline with the promise to help you "lose weight quickly" or "get ready for summer" but with *the catch* in fine print to just follow these rules, eliminate these food groups, and take these fat-burning supplements. Never mind what our body actually needs, right? Let's just get the weight off fast! Then we are exhausted from counting every carb gram and we miss our favorite foods. We just have to hope and pray we don't burn out and give up and gain all the weight back. That is such an exhausting way to live! Can I get an amen?

I myself used to live this way. I lost touch of what my body needed, and I dove headfirst into calorie counting and eliminating all the "bad foods" in order to lose weight. Do you want to know what happened? Because my body was no longer getting the proper nutrients and specifically enough fat and carb sources it needed to create enough cholesterol, my hormones shut down. Or should I say, specifically, my menstrual cycle completely stopped for six months and I ended up suffering from severe depression, anxiety, and mood swings as a result. Hormones have so much influence on our mental health and when they become imbalanced, we suffer, often in more ways than one. I had always been a bubbly, happy girl. Depression and anxiety just weren't in my vocabulary. Until one day, they were.

You see, my body no longer had what it needed to fuel itself properly and it ended up in survival mode. I ended up seeing my doctor and he ordered blood work. Low and behold, my progesterone and estrogen were in the basement, along with my iron. If you don't already know, you need a certain amount of cholesterol and nutrients to make each of these hormones in order to have a normal menstrual cycle and to stay happy and anxiety-free. You also need enough healthy fats and B vitamins to create mood-balancing neurotransmitters such as serotonin and dopamine. Basically, when in survival mode, one of the first things to go on the back burner is our reproductive system, followed by our mental stability. After months of working hard to nourish my body back to health, my menstrual cycle finally returned. However, the depression and anxiety lingered, and it lingered for years. The hormones fluctuating as they did triggered a chemical imbalance in my brain and it has unfortunately taken me until this past year to start feeling like myself again. Hormone imbalances are no joke.

I realized after going through this very rough period in my life that even though I had lost the weight I had wanted to, I had punished my body and paid an extremely steep price that I hadn't bargained for. Now, perhaps you can relate. Perhaps you also have caused your body stress and strain at some point by trying to walk on a tightrope for a different reason. Perhaps your body reacted totally differently than mine did. Our stories don't have to be the same for us to understand each other. We all know there have been times we have pushed ourselves over the edge and we have ended up regretting it. In the end, though, every trial in life results in a new life lesson learned. We end up coming out stronger than we went in and so for that, I am grateful.

This dark period in my life is actually what persuaded me to start studying nutrition and what eventually drove me to get certified as a nutrition and wellness consultant through the American Fitness Professionals Association (AFPA) nearly ten years ago now. I thought to myself, "There just has to be another way to stay in shape, maintain my weight, and feel amazing both mentally and physically!" Through my healing process, I eventually discovered the truth that has led me to where I am today. *If you start something extreme and expect your body to jump through hoops like some circus animal in order to hit a goal, your body WILL eventually suffer and have negative effects to show from it.* You will eventually burn out and you will eventually lose touch with your body and your healthy relationship with food. Food will become a burden to you instead of something to be enjoyed, and you will wish you could go back and do it all over again. Trust me, I sure regret what I put my body through.

So please, hear me out. If you are being told that you have to eliminate an entire food group, eat all of your food in a four-hour window, and count every single calorie or carb gram, then run for the hills as fast as you can. What I teach and the lifestyle I live by can be implemented at home, at work, or on vacation and you can put it into practice *forever*. My message to you is simply this. Before dipping your toes into anything seemingly healthy or weight-loss focused, ask yourself this one question: "Can I do this every single day for the rest of my life?" If the answer is yes, then go for it! If the answer is no, then walk (or run) away. *Remember, if it sounds too good to be true, it probably is.* Your body doesn't want to lose ten pounds in one week on a liquid diet. It wants to be cared for and given all the nutrients it needs.

Do yourself a favor and don't just eat the bare minimum to get by. We don't want to just be barely making it, do we? No! We want to be able to breeze through our day and have energy to spare at the end of it! Lastly, please don't ever take out an entire food group in an attempt to shed some unwanted pounds. Our body needs protein, fat, carbohydrates, fruits and veggies, and lots and lots of water to be at its best. It needs it *all*! Just fuel your body properly and give it all that it needs and it will all just click! You will feel energetic, happy, and full of life. Then real weight loss that lasts will become a natural side effect. So my message to you is this: *love on your body and it will love on you!*

Principle Two: *Discover The 80/20 Lifestyle And Then Live By It*

If you have followed me on my blog or social media for any period of time, then you will have heard by now about this 80/20 ratio that I swear and live by. I can honestly tell you that it wasn't until I discovered how vital this ratio was that I truly felt free around food again and I stopped being afraid of my cravings. Nowadays, I eat whatever I want, and I am in better shape and health than I was ten years ago before having kids! The catch is that I do it mindfully and I implement this ratio into how I eat every single day. I can have everything I want, just in moderation.

The beauty of this lifestyle is it naturally takes away any and all stress one may have around food and it helps take care of your cravings and any feelings of deprivation. It is broken down like this: *80 percent of the time, I make it a point to eat whole foods that are grown from the earth, which are not processed and are void of gluten, refined sugar, meat, and dairy. Then, 20 percent of the time, I leave room for anything I want to eat regardless of how it is made or what is in it.* If I really want something, I make sure to include it in that 20 percent of my day or week and I don't have any guilt about it whatsoever.

It all comes down to being honest with yourself and taking a moment to evaluate how you really eat. Are you more on the lines of fifty-fifty? Ask yourself this and answer honestly. Then, make the appropriate adjustments until you have reached a ratio of 80/20. The easiest way I have found to implement this ratio is to allow for *one small treat a day*. I usually stick to dark chocolate, but if I want a brownie, I have a brownie. If I want some ice cream, then I have some. I indulge in what sounds good, but I try and keep it small. Without fail, though, I have something sweet *every* single day.

Then, once a week, I recommend having what I call a "20 meal" or a "splurge meal" (*not* an entire day) where I can enjoy *whatever* my taste buds desire! Believe it or not, allowing your body to indulge like this actually challenges your metabolism and encourages it to burn even more efficiently for up to seventy-two hours! Have you ever found yourself extremely hungry the day after Thanksgiving? Well, now you know why. Think of it this way. If you fuel your body with the exact same amount of food each and every day, eventually it will get used to it and your metabolism will not have to work as hard. One of the biggest things I see is that plateaus seem to happen the most when our body is underfed or is being fed without any variation. That is why those fifteen hundred meal plans only work for so long. So think of your "20 meal" as pouring kerosene on your bonfire. *By allowing yourself this freedom to indulge once a week, you are actually encouraging your body to burn fat and calories even more efficiently for you!* How fascinating is that?

Now for me, I have honestly found that at this stage of motherhood, I just don't enjoy indulging when my kids are around because I am mentally still in "mom mode" and not able to fully relax and focus on my food. Aside from that, more times than not, my little ones think that whatever I am eating is up for grabs, so I generally only end up eating a few bites of it. This is not to sound resentful in any way. It is just the stage of life that I am in with little ones running around. Needless to say, I leave my treat for when my kids go to bed each night and I leave my "20 meal for when I go out to eat on a date with my husband or girlfriends or for an event such as a wedding or work party. This way, I can really enjoy every bite and focus on what I am eating. Who wants to indulge in a yummy meal and not be able to fully enjoy it? Not this momma!

Now back to this "20 meal. I firmly believe this *has* to happen weekly in order to maintain a lifestyle and not feel as if you are on a diet. Why is this? Well, I've said it before and I will say it again. Diets and deprivation do *not* work and they are not maintainable. You have to have the freedom to some degree to go out and enjoy what you love. Not to say that I don't fully enjoy healthy food because I so do! But there is just something so liberating about being able to sit down at a restaurant and order whatever I want without feeling guilty. Let me tell you, on date night I have been known to out eat my husband (true story). Give me the breadsticks, spaghetti carbonara with extra bacon bits, wine, and tiramisu and I am one happy girl!

Now, as you may have picked up on, I do not believe in calling this a "cheat meal." Why is this? Because "cheating," to me, has negative connotations. It implies that I am doing something wrong when indeed I am *not*. I am just living my best life and enjoying what I love in moderation! Could there be any better way to live? I think not!

Principle Three: *If You Aren't A Planner Then Become One*

A healthy life doesn't just happen. As with anything worthwhile in life, it requires strategic *planning*. Let me help you get started with these basic questions first. What foods do I want into my body? What recipes do I want to make this coming week? When am I going to the grocery store? When am I going to meal prep or take the time to cook these recipes? Time and time again as a nutritional consultant, I have heard that "I just don't have time to eat healthy or lead a healthy life." The truth is we are all busy. No one has the luxury of zero responsibilities. Whether you are a full-time employee, a stay-at-home-mom, a working mom from home, or are retired, I think it is safe to say we all have things going on and keeping us very busy.

So what gives? How can we possibly find extra time to grocery shop and cook healthy snacks and meals for ourselves and for our families? The answer is simple. We have to *make* the time but first, start by making our health a high enough priority. The truth is it really doesn't take as much time as you think. Practically speaking, it takes on average twenty to thirty minutes to meal plan for the week ahead, twenty to thirty minutes to write a grocery list based off that meal plan, one or two hours to grocery shop (or even less if you choose to order on your phone and have it delivered), maybe thirty extra minutes to an hour of baking on the weekend, and twenty minutes an evening to throw together a wholesome meal.

That may sound like a lot, but truthfully it isn't when you consider that there are twenty-four hours in a day and 168 hours in a week. On average, that is only four hours a week, total, that we need to set aside to feed our families and ourselves well. We can *all* do that! Now, before you start thinking of all of the reasons this can't work for you, take a minute and ask yourself how important living a long life is to you. Remember, food can be the best form of medicine or the worst form of poison. When we are feeding it processed, inflammatory foods all day long, what can we expect? The answer is a lot of health issues, trouble maintaining a healthy weight, and more.

Why are prepackaged meal services so popular these days? Because all of the work is done for you. Now, though I am in no way against using them from time to time, I think that if we are relying on a food service or prepackaged meals of any sort to fuel us, then we are hurting our relationship with food *and* our kitchen. There is something so rewarding and fulfilling about cooking up nourishing food in our own kitchen. We get to focus and think about every single ingredient going into our meal and into our bodies. We also get to appreciate the taste even more because we know that *we* created it.

Lastly, taking the time to plan our meals and make them ourselves gives us more confidence in the kitchen and it shows us that we are capable of caring for our bodies and families without having to rely on a pricey food service. If you have little ones in your home, they are also looking up to you and seeing you in the kitchen and unknowingly are building their confidence as well. So my suggestion to you is this. Purchase a pretty meal planner if you don't already have one and start meal planning away. I promise you it is not as intimidating as you think! Plan and then plan some more! That is the only way to make a healthy lifestyle a reality. If I can do it, you can do it. Trust me on this!

Principle Four: *Just Eat Real Food*

I am always amazed to think back on how my tiny five-foot-tall grandmother used to cook and eat. I remember she used to butter everything and bake everything you could think of under the sun. I remember walking into her house when we would come to visit and there would be an array of delicious food on her table just waiting for us. Her coconut cake and homemade macaroni and cheese were also my favorite! She made everything from scratch and she made sure every ingredient was fresh. She made and ate everything her heart desired in moderation. Let me emphasize again that nearly everything this tiny and healthy woman ate was *real and unprocessed.* She also focused on eating every food group, which I am a firm believer in as well. Our body *thrives* off being fed a balanced diet! It is vital that we include lean or plant-based protein, healthy fat sources from avocados, coconut oil, real butter, nuts, and other plant oils, as well as gluten-free, whole-grain carbohydrates, and also an array of colorful fruits and veggies all throughout our day!

You see, when we consistently fuel our body this way, it gets what it needs to function properly, it can give us back the energy we need to go about our day, *and* it keeps our metabolism at its prime. Our culture focuses so much on calories in and calories out. I hate to break it to you, but calories really don't mean as much as you may think. Calories basically represent a unit of energy. But what they don't tell us is how our body processes that specific form of fuel and how it can benefit our body or wear it down.

A bag of potato chips, for instance, in comparison to a steamed sweet potato with a tablespoon of real butter on top, may equal about the same number of calories, but they both affect our bodies completely differently. Potato chips have been linked to weight gain and an array of health issues such as high blood pressure and even cancer, but a buttered sweet potato has been shown to burn belly fat due to its high fiber content, protects our bodies against cancer, and reduces inflammation due to its high vitamin and antioxidant content.

So I will say it again. *Our body wants to be fed food it can easily recognize.* When we take in food such as potato chips that have been processed in a factory, preserved, and then bathed in excess bleached salt, our body isn't happy with us. Our taste buds may be for the time being, but in reality, we aren't doing ourselves any favors. Our body doesn't just simply utilize and dispose of processed food. Instead, our body recognizes processed foods and additives as foreign and it responds with inflammation, water retention, and fat gain due to the high glycemic index (which is a recipe for a blood sugar spike followed by a crash). Inflammation of any sort can suppress the thyroid gland, and the thyroid gland controls our metabolism. So, do the math.

Processed foods are mostly void of nutrition, so they require little energy burn to break them down. On the other hand, whole foods, ironically, require our body to burn *more* energy in order to break them down and distribute the nutrients throughout our body. The difference is we aren't left with yucky health effects in the end, and we end up storing less energy or fat because more calories were actually burned during the digestion process. So, when we eat whole foods, we actually are turning our body into a calorie- and fat-burning machine. How cool is that? Also, thanks to the high fiber content and nutrient make-up found in whole foods, they do a great job keeping our blood sugar stable, which is one of the number-one ways to stay in the fat-burning zone all day long. Not to mention, whole foods keep us fuller for much longer and keep us from becoming "hangry." We all know how much fun that is!

Now, though I do not believe in ever removing an entire food group, I do recommend *limiting* dairy and gluten and keeping them in your 20 window. This is because they both have been linked to inflammation, digestive upset, eczema, acne, weight gain, and more. They have also been shown to cause flareups in those with autoimmune diseases, making their symptoms even more profound. That being said, some of my favorite dairy alternatives are coconut, almond or oat milk or yogurt, and some of my favorite gluten alternatives are brown or wild rice and quinoa, oats, natural popcorn, almond flour, coconut flour, and sweet potatoes. You will see in some of my recipes I use a small amount of butter or a small amount of cheese, but again, I don't exclude either dairy or gluten from my diet completely (again, this is a lifestyle and NOT a cookie-cutter diet). I just try to keep my consumption of them minimal because I have seen in both myself and in many others what a difference it can make in overall health. I really believe that if you focus on only consuming them in moderation, you will notice many positive changes as well.

So remember, many whole foods may be calorically equivalent to many processed or inflammatory foods, but they are metabolized and put to use in *very* different ways within the body. As a nutritional consultant for nearly nine years, I have witnessed firsthand how much this is true in men and women of all ages. I have also seen this in myself as I for sure used to eat way less in a day but in the form of frozen, low-calorie meals and one-hundred-calorie snack packs (yuck!). Whereas now, I can tell you that I eat significantly more than I used to but in the form of real, whole foods (80 percent of the time), and I am in the best shape of my life even after having my babies. All that to say, I am a passionate believer in eating real, whole foods that nourish our bodies and I hope you are as well—or will soon be the further you go in this book!

Principle Five: *Eat Small But Eat Often*

Now this one requires us to put our planning skills into practice like we just talked about. If you want to lose weight and really keep it off long-term, then this principle, along with focusing primarily on eating whole foods, is extremely important. Allow me to explain why.

Our metabolism (or the rate at which our body burns calories), is like a bonfire. It requires kindling all day long in order to keep the flame burning. *One of the worst ways to sabotage our metabolism is by skipping meals or going too long in general without eating on a routine basis.* Just try and think back to when you were a child. You, like most children, probably ate a little here and a little there all throughout the day. Kids rarely sit and devour a whole plate of food and stuff themselves. Instead, they eat small, but they eat often. This is the way we should all still be eating, but unfortunately, this way of eating is often forgotten by the time the teenage years hit when our parents are no longer helicoptering over us and serving us every meal and snack.

I remember back in high school when I started forgetting to eat. I was usually running late to school, so a bite of a white bagel was sometimes all I had time for in the morning and then I would usually grab cookies out of the vending machine if I forgot lunch a few hours later when I started to crash. Then, when I got home, I would heat up some pizza bites and binge a couple of hours later at dinner. Then I would wake up and do it all over again.

Then fast-forward to my freshman year of college and my first year of marriage when my eating habits started tanking even more. I have a distinct memory of one day rushing to class and being too busy to eat (again) and just grabbing a Tootsie Roll out of a candy jar in the front office. That Tootsie Roll was the only thing I ate that day until dinner. I wish I was making this up, but I'm not. What I ate was just an afterthought at that time in my life. Did I mention that I am also hypoglycemic and am prone to low blood sugar as it is? I just cringe thinking back to those days. I was jittery and I had trouble focusing and honestly felt like garbage. Any time I did manage to eat a normal diet, perhaps on the weekends, I noticed that I would see it instantly on the scale.

When I got married at the age of eighteen, I had unknowingly already damaged my metabolism and asked it to function at a snail's pace. When I moved in with my husband and started relaxing and eating more fast food and garbage like him *and* started a desk job as a receptionist, what do you think happened? You guessed it. I instantly put on twelve pounds. Now, twelve pounds may not sound astronomical to you, but for someone who is five foot one inch tall, twelve pounds matter a whole heck of a lot.

You may be reading this and thinking, "You were only eighteen. Didn't you have youth on your side?" This misconception is one that I hear the most. I have parents contact me concerned over their teen and unsure as to why they at "their young age" are struggling so much with their weight. Then I also have elderly clients contact me, asking if there is anything they can really do to lose weight "at their old age." Of course, then there are those I have talked with who feel discouraged by their family history of obesity and assume they must be doomed. *You may find it encouraging to learn that I actually think quite the opposite. Without a doubt, it is my belief that our metabolism is still very much in our control despite our age and our genetics. I will acknowledge that they play a small part, yes, but what and how often we feed our body can absolutely help to persuade our metabolism to work in our favor (or against us) regardless of who we are or what stage of life we are in.*

When I first was studying nutrition, I wanted to know if there was anything I could possibly do to fix my metabolism and rev it back up to its full capacity again. Was there even any hope left for me after the past few years I had spent telling my metabolism to slow down? The answer was a resounding *yes!* I am here to tell you that if you are asking yourself the same question today, there is always hope and it is never too late! If you are in the same boat today as I was ten years ago or as many of my clients are when they first come into my office, then I want to encourage you that you *can* reverse the damage and get your metabolism working in your favor once again!

Now, that all sounds great, but how does one go about doing this and in a practical way? The answer is simple. *We must fuel our body regularly again by remembering one, two, and three.*

- **Eat within ONE hour of waking up.** This is so important because no matter how fast your metabolism runs during the day, it settles down for the night when you settle down. It does not know to rev back up to its daytime pace until you first put food in your mouth.
- **Eat every TWO and no more than three hours during the day.** Remember that bonfire we were talking about? Our body needs to be fueled often to keep that fire going and to keep our body in fat-burning mode all day long. When it thinks that there isn't sufficient food around, it slows down as a protective mechanism.
- **Stop eating THREE hours before bedtime (unless you are a diabetic or are told otherwise by your doctor).** Why would you fill up a car with a full tank of gas only to sit still in a parking lot? Though our body is still burning *some* calories while sleeping, it burns them more efficiently during the day when we are up moving around. So, if you go to bed around 11 p.m. like I do, then make it a point to finish your last meal or snack around 8 p.m. It's as easy as that! Avoiding eating close to bedtime also helps give your digestive tract a break and time to process any remaining food from the day, ensuring a flatter belly when you wake up, with less

bloat and less chance of constipation. Now again, don't forget the 80/20 lifestyle we talked about. Most nights I aim for a three-hour gap before bed, but once or twice a week it may be closer to one or two hours before bed. Remember, a lifestyle isn't about perfection. It leaves wiggle room for you to enjoy life and relax a little, and that, to me, is a beautiful thing!

This way of eating is known as "grazing." It's *not* a diet. It can be done anywhere and everyone can do it! Even many individuals with a medical diagnosis such as hypothyroidism or diabetes can benefit and boost their metabolism when they incorporate grazing into their lives. Trust me, I've seen it many times and I can tell you that it really works! Later in this book, I will be providing you with a sample five-day meal plan to help get you started, so just be on the lookout for that.

So, do you want to know how to gauge if your metabolism is finally speeding up and working in your favor? It is simple. *You will notice that you are a little more hungry a little more often. This is a telltale sign that your body is burning the food you feed it efficiently!* I have clients that tell me they used to be able to go all day without eating or even thinking about food and now when the two- or three-hour mark hits they HAVE to eat! This change in hunger cues isn't a mystery. It is simply due to the fact that you let your body know there is abundant food around and that it is no longer required to go hours running on empty. Your body will no longer be in survival mode, where it feels the need to hold on for dear life to every bite of food you give it as a means to survive. It now will be relaxed and happy and once again burning efficiently for you! Cheers to that!

Principle Six: *Stop Counting Calories and Just Grab A Salad Plate*

In addition to the grazing lifestyle, we really have to keep portion control in mind. *When we implement grazing into our daily routine, the key is to eat twice as often but half as much at each meal.* Did you know that your stomach is about the size of your fist? It's not a very large organ at all. Unfortunately, what so often happens when we skip meals is that we end up overeating later and stretching our stomach. Our stomach is flexible like a rubber band. When we overfill it, it can be stretched over time, therefore leaving us feeling deprived even after eating a normal amount of food. On the other hand, with proper portion control, we have the ability to shrink our stomach back to its original size and once again be satisfied with a smaller, more appropriate amount of food.

So this is where the "salad plate principle" comes in. The idea is this. If everything we eat can fit on a salad plate, then we won't be able to stretch our stomach. When I first learned of this relaxed method of portion control years ago, I thought it was brilliant. It took out all of the stress and anxiety of guessing all day if I was eating too much or too little. I quickly put it into practice and began teaching it to all of my clients. The beauty is we don't need to count every calorie or carb gram, weigh or measure our food, and obsess over every bite we eat. We just have to be able to recognize what a salad-plate-size portion of food looks like and, of course, aim to eat as balanced as possible *and* include protein, fat, carbohydrates at every meal, and also incorporate colorful fruits and veggies throughout our day as well.

If we stick to smaller, more frequent portions of food, it is nearly impossible to stretch our stomachs. Did you know that one hundred years ago the average size of a dinner plate was the size of our salad plate today? Our dinner plates have grown over two inches in size and so have the majority of our waistlines! Now, obviously, it is not always possible to eat every meal or snack on a salad plate, but if you try to do so as often as possible, then you will eventually learn what a proper portion looks like and won't need one to gauge it. One trick I have up my sleeve is that when I am out to eat, I ask the server for a box and put half away for later *before* I am tempted to eat the whole entrée. Most American restaurants serve about three times the proper portion in one entrée, so always try and put half away for later.

Now, oftentimes when I teach this old-fashioned principle to my clients, they quickly fire back at first with how hungry they would be if they only ate a salad-plate amount of food. What they are forgetting though, is that they are now eating every two or three hours! Eating often keeps us from getting to the point of feeling uncomfortably hungry and jittery and grabbing any food within our reach as a quick fix. Typically when our blood sugar plummets, we end up craving carbs and sugar and that, my friends, is where the "3 p.m. slump" and the junk food binging hour comes in. When we graze, however, we come to the dinner table calm, cool, and collected, ready to enjoy and savor a healthy portion of food. We are not ravenous, and we have the ability to control ourselves and not overdo it.

We are no longer "starving" or "stuffed." We are just satisfied and our stomach feels flatter than it has in years and our digestive tract is also happier and running more efficiently. We are eating small and often and now our blood sugar is stable and we no longer crash at 3 p.m. and have to army crawl to the vending machine for a pick-me-up. Our pants are fitting better and we are eating more than we used to. Bizarre, isn't it? You see, this is how I believe our bodies were intended to be fed. THIS is what the Live Healthy With Laura lifestyle is all about. It is about feeling satisfied, well-nourished, energetic, and full of life all day long!

So, next time you are about to serve yourself a meal, reach for that salad plate. If you want more, you can always have more later if you really want to! Keep in mind though that it takes your brain a full twenty minutes to register that you ate a meal or snack. So, watch that clock and don't jump to grab seconds unless it has been a full twenty minutes! Your brain may just not have gotten the cue that you've been fed yet! Now, of course, there will be days when you have been more physically active or (if you are a woman) PMS decides to show up, or for some unknown reason you just find yourself unusually hungry. Listen to those cues and please don't ignore them! Tune in and listen to your body. This is a very important part of a healthy lifestyle, which we will touch more on in the next chapter.

Now, I have to shine light once more on the 80/20 lifestyle because, again, I don't want you to aim for perfection in *any* area, this area included. If I am being honest, sometimes I myself will overeat. If it is my treasured 20 night, for instance, and I am out on a date with my husband or out with girlfriends, then sometimes I will just polish off that bowl of pasta and scarf down a breadstick too. Then, of course, I love a glass or two of wine, and dessert always ends up sounding good too, so I will typically order that as well. I could blame it on the wine or the fact that I get a little too excited to have an adult-only night out, but it all comes down to one thing. I am human. Do I feel bloated and a bit rundown afterwards? I sure do. But real life allows for setbacks. *Most* of the time I try and leave with a box, but once in a while I don't, and that's okay too.

One thing I no longer do is beat myself up about it anymore like I used to. I don't feel the need to go for a run after I indulge, or starve myself the next day. I instead acknowledge that again, I am human, and I give myself credit for the fact that for the majority of the time, I eat clean and practice portion control. So what if I give myself a little wiggle room? A lifestyle is about balance, and what matters the most is what you do in that 80 percent window. Give yourself that 20 percent to breathe and let go a little! If you do, on occasion, overeat, then just regroup the next day and start fresh. *Give yourself grace.* This is essential for a healthy mind and body!

Principle Seven: *Tune Into Your Body*

Our body is constantly trying to communicate with us. God gave our bodies the amazing ability to recognize a need and relay the message quickly to our brains so that we can then respond accordingly. What unfortunately so often happens though in this hectic world we live in, is that these messages often get ignored and pushed under the rug. If we are tired, instead of going to bed earlier, we just drink another cup of coffee. If we are stressed out, we don't say no to another obligation and give ourselves a much-needed break, but instead, we push ourselves even harder. If we are hungry, we often don't take the time to stop and eat. If we do, we grab something quick and convenient. We do so without thinking if that meal or snack is doing anything beneficial for us. Later, when we finally get around to sitting down for dinner after a long day, we tend to overdo it, and we don't stop to evaluate if our body has had enough.

Our body is always trying to reach a state of homeostasis, yet we are constantly working against it. We then wonder why in the world we are walking around feeling depleted and cranky and unable to lose weight. Did you know that when our body is constantly under stress and not being properly cared for, our cortisol or our "fight or flight hormone" stays elevated? Instead of it being released when we have to run from someone trying to rob us in a parking lot, it is constantly secreted all day long. We keep trying to go full speed on the treadmill of life. Because of this, our body not only holds on to fat more easily (in case it thinks we need to run for our lives again); it also suppresses our metabolism in order to conserve enough energy for us to run away. It may sound bizarre, but this is what high cortisol communicates to the brain. Have you ever wondered why you can go on vacation, not workout at all, indulge a bit more, yet not gain a single pound? You guessed it. Your body is relaxed and happy, and your cortisol is finally back to a healthy level!

Allow me to help you understand tuning into your body from a different angle. Ask yourself if you would tell a six-month-old baby under your care to just "stop crying" or to just "suck it up." Of course you wouldn't do that. Yet, so often we say this to ourselves time and time again. If our baby was crying we would instantly stop what we were doing and figure out what it needed, right? So then why do we treat our bodies any differently than we would a child? It all comes down to the fact that *we* are no longer a high enough priority to ourselves. We give and give so much of ourselves, yet many of us have lost touch of who we are and what we need.

I want to be as transparent with you as possible and tell you that until I got my anxiety and depression under control (by the grace of God and with both Western and holistic medicine, combined) I had my share of very scary panic attacks. Ironically enough, those panic attacks seemed to always pop up when I was feeling most out of tune with my body and overtaxed in more ways than one. I am grateful to say that now I can recognize when burnout is coming and when my body needs a break. It took me a long time to get to where I am today, but my rocky journey is what inspired me to write this book to hopefully help you avoid some of the rough patches I had to go through and to help encourage you to start making yourself a priority once again.

We must stop making ourselves an afterthought. Tune in to your body and start by sitting down and asking yourself these questions:

1. On a scale of 1-10, what is my average stress level on an average day?
2. On a scale of 1-10, what is my energy level throughout the day? Do I have a crashing point? (If you get tired all of a sudden around 3 p.m., your adrenal glands may be taxed, but we will touch on that in the next chapter.)

3. How much sleep did I get last night and how do I feel today?
4. What did I eat last and how did it make me feel twenty minutes later?
5. When did I last eat? Am I hungry now?
6. How much water have I drunk today? How much water did I drink yesterday?
7. Do I have any cravings today? If so, what are they?
8. How do I feel when I am around food (guilty, stressed, relaxed, or joyful)?
9. When is the last time I gave myself a day off from any optional responsibilities?
10. When is the last time I gave myself a few hours to do something I enjoy?
11. What is my favorite way to exercise and how often do I move my body in this way?
12. How many commitments do I have and what can I let go of?

Do you see what I mean? We need to be in constant communication with ourselves and always be asking questions. Keep a journal or a log in your phone with how you feel each and every week. Make sure to record any new stressors that come into play as well. When we tune in like this, we have the chance to evaluate how we are *really* feeling. We aren't letting weeks of self-neglect build up that result in a panic attack or burnout, because we are constantly checking in. If something is feeling "off," we then can acknowledge it and show our body love by making the proper adjustments until we feel healthy and happy again. This applies to our mental, spiritual, and physical health. They all connect and keep us balanced! So, if it has been a while since you've tuned in and checked on yourself (and not just everyone else), then I want to encourage you to please do that *today*.

Principle Eight: *Remember, You Are What You DRINK*

With so much hype about what we are eating, I think it's about time to bring up one very important topic: *what we drink.* So often, I will come across a friend or a client who says to me, "Laura, I'm eating so well and exercising regularly, yet I can't drop a single pound!" I totally can understand how frustrating it must be when someone feels as if they are putting in so much time and effort, only to come out empty-handed. If I was meeting with you in person today, the first thing I would do is hand you a questionnaire that would walk me through your day and through your lifestyle habits. I would ask you to write down everything you eat and drink on a daily basis and everything you ate and drank yesterday, specifically. What I so often find is that many people are already trying to make healthier food choices by the time they start consulting with me, but their beverages stick out to me like a big red flag.

So many beverages we drink and ingredients that we add to our beverages are actually hidden sugar and chemical bombs. As you know, a high amount of refined sugar is a recipe for weight gain and fat retention. Not to mention, it feeds cancer and causes inflammation all throughout the body, suppresses our immune system, makes us look older by breaking down our collagen, and leaves us in the dump later, after we come off our sugar high. Did you know that some coffee creamers contain just about the same amount of sugar as a candy bar and those that are "sugar-free" often contain tons of additives and chemicals (in fine print, of course)? Now, don't even get me started on soda or those five-dollar Frappuccinos or Macchiatos so many of us so easily get hooked on. I am not saying they are not okay every once in a while as a treat (anything can be incorporated in the 80/20 lifestyle), but just keep in mind that you aren't doing your health any favors if you drink them daily.

So what about juice? It may surprise you to learn that that glass of orange juice you just chugged this morning actually spiked your blood sugar twice as fast as a whole, freshly peeled orange would have. This goes for green juices and many popular detox smoothies as well. Juice does contain a natural form of sugar, however, the glycemic index (the rate at which it affects our body's blood sugar) is much higher and it also loses most of its glucose-stabilizing fiber content in the juicing process. So, totally enjoy juice on occasion, but just keep this in mind. Whole, untampered-with fruits and veggies will always give you more bang for your buck.

Now, I can't move on without bringing up alcoholic beverages. There are ways that you can drink alcohol in moderation and still keep your health in check. However, I will just tell you that *I have seen most people struggle with their weight and belly fat specifically when they are having more than two alcoholic beverages a week on average.* This could be due to the fact that alcohol in general increases estrogen and high estrogen increases belly fat, or it could be due to the sugar content in the type of alcohol you are drinking. Alcohol can also wear and tear on your liver when drunk in excess, so keep that in mind too. Now listen, I personally love my wine on a night out on the town or on a Friday night after a long week and I don't plan on ever giving it up! However, going back to the Live Healthy With Laura motto, I practice *moderation* with everything I eat or drink and I keep my wine or any alcoholic beverages in the 20 percent category. I consider it a treat, and I definitely don't recommend it becoming a daily habit.

After discussing all of the above, I'm sure you have been waiting to see when I would finally bring up coffee. Don't worry. I could never forget about my favorite morning ritual. I savor my morning cup of coffee as soon as I get up (after a big glass of water), with a splash of coconut milk and a dash of monk fruit or stevia, but *not*, however, with a sugary, artificially flavored creamer of any sort. I make sure to keep all of the ingredients clean, but I am a *huge* coffee fan and I never go a day without it! After all, I am a mommy whose children's sleep patterns are very unpredictable and a blogger who often finds herself up a bit too late at night. Even before I ever became a parent or started blogging, though, I was madly in love with coffee. I love the cozy aroma and the mood and energy boost it gives me each morning. In addition to how it makes me feel and how amazing it smells, coffee is loaded with antioxidants and it helps lower our risk for Alzheimer's, heart disease, and some forms of cancer. So with all of that said, naturally, I feel that it is a win-win! But of course, as with anything, too much of a good thing can end up becoming an issue and causing problems.

Coffee (and caffeine of any form) is a stimulant, meaning it stimulates our central nervous system. It helps us to perk up in the mornings and get going for the day. *But* what happens when we drink coffee or caffeine all throughout the day? Well, for starters, we end up feeling anxious and jittery and we tend to struggle with insomnia later when it's time to go to sleep. Then on the next level, too much caffeine for an extended period of time causes our adrenal glands (the little thumb-sized glands above our kidneys) to go into overdrive. What happens then? You guessed it. We soon crash, and we crash hard! We may be able to slide by with a few weeks or even months of consuming an overload of caffeine before we realize it's caused an issue. But trust me, if it hasn't already, your body will let you know soon that it isn't happy. Adrenal fatigue isn't pretty and it can leave us feeling "wired but tired," panicky, depressed, forgetful, and it can also result in unwanted weight gain. None of this sounds appealing now, does it? *This is why I recommend having only one cup of coffee or caffeinated beverage before lunchtime and that's it.* This will allow us to receive a boost without taxing our body in the meantime and having to pay the price later.

Okay, so what about if we aren't really drinking any sugary beverages, loads of coffee, or an abundance of alcohol, but we also aren't drinking much of anything at all? Well, as much as I hate to be the bearer of bad news, I have to tell you that this is *just* as detrimental to your health and waistline! I speak to clients often who somehow manage to get through their day with only a few sips of water here and there (this makes me thirsty just thinking about it!) This is so harmful and taxing on the body. Our body depends so much on water! It keeps our body functioning in more ways than one.

When we don't drink enough water, our body can't burn fat properly, fight infection properly, or detox efficiently. *Our body is made up of 70 percent water and we need to drink half of our body weight in ounces a day in order to stay properly hydrated!* This sounds like a lot, and it is, but when we start from the moment we wake up and keep it with us at arm's reach all day, it ends up being very doable! The average American woman for instance, weighs 170 pounds. So that is eighty-five ounces of water or close to three liters of water a day. It is not as overwhelming as you may think. Again, it is all about making it a priority and making sure it is at arm's reach *all day long!* Once you start properly hydrating your body, you will start to crave water and it will no longer be such a hassle.

I highly suggest you do yourself a favor and purchase a large one-liter bottle as soon as you are able. Trust me when I say that you will find that it is *much* easier to get enough H2O in your day when you aren't constantly having to get up and refill your glass constantly. Who really has time for that, anyways? Lastly, do your best to avoid drinking out of plastics (as they can wreak havoc on your hormone balance) and stick to drinking out of glass or stainless steel as much as possible.

All this being said, the point that I am trying to make is simply that you can't be at your healthiest and most fit without drinking enough water. You just can't. It really is essential for a vibrant, energetic, and thriving body. So, if you are one of the many who do not drink enough water, then I urge you to work hard and really focus on getting enough in. You will be *amazed* by how much better you look and feel when you are properly hydrated. You also might just discover that it was the missing link holding you back from reaching your full health potential!

Principle Nine: *Sleep Like It's Going Out Of Style*

Let me be honest and start off by saying that I rarely deprive myself of much of anything, but sleep seems to be the first thing to go when I am under a lot of pressure, or I am at my busiest. I am sure I am not alone in this. With so much going on in all of our lives, it is easy to try and skimp on as little sleep as possible to seemingly have more hours in our day. I have to tell you, though, that when I miss out on sleep, I *always* regret it. It affects my mind and body so much and it does yours as well, even if you don't realize it. *An adult requires between seven to nine hours of solid sleep a night to function properly.* Scientifically, sleep is proven to help us "reset" in about a million different ways but more specifically it:

- balances our hormones (both thyroid and sex hormones)
- reduces our stress hormone, cortisol
- boosts our immunity
- boosts our metabolism and encourages our bodies to burn fat (you snooze, you literally lose!)
- improves our digestion and blood circulation (goodbye constipation!)
- stabilizes our blood sugar
- lowers inflammation in the body (think glowing skin, less joint pain, and a lower risk for cancer and diseases)
- lowers our risk of heart attack and stroke
- reduces anxiety and depression and improves overall mental health

... and more! So needless to say, sleep really isn't optional if we want to reach and maintain our FULL health potential!

But what if you can't get enough sleep because you feel you have too much to do? What if you can't sleep because you have too much on your mind? How much sleep do you actually need to be at your best?

Allow me to simplify and break down all of the sleep questions and dilemmas you may have:

- If you are going to bed late and waking up early, then you are burning the candle at both ends. Decide what you can take off your plate because something *has* to give and it can*not* be your sleep.
- If you are going to bed on time but can't seem to fall asleep, then consider journaling your thoughts before bed and also using topical magnesium oil before bed (of course, after consulting with your physician).
- If you work with screens in the evening or a lot during the day, then I highly recommend purchasing blue-light glasses. Blue light from screens of any form disrupts our circadian rhythm at night by preventing melatonin (our sleep hormone) from being appropriately produced.
- Aim to unwind at least thirty minutes before bed and stop anything that requires your brain to do extra work. Pick a book that is uplifting to read in those last thirty minutes, but do your best to stay off social media, the news, checking your email, or anything work-related.
- Take a warm bath before bed and light some candles (when you have the extra time, of course).
- Dim the lights or turn off as many lights as possible after dinnertime to help calm your mind and body and to help it produce more melatonin.
- Consider purchasing blackout curtains to help keep your room as dark as possible from morning to night.

With all of these in mind, I just want to encourage you to do whatever you possibly can to get adequate amounts of sleep each night. Try these tips and experiment to see what works for you. When you make sleep a high priority, your body and mind will thank you immensely! Remember, there will always be something that can get in the way of our sleep *if* we let it. Let's remember the value of sleep and stop being willing to sacrifice it. Let's sleep our way to a healthier mind and physique together, shall we? Our body does so much for us. It is the least we can do to help it recharge!

Principle Ten: *Move The Way Your Body Wants To Move*

For those of you who detest exercise, I have some news I think you will be happy to hear. What you eat is *really* what matters the most! You simply can't outrun a bad diet (so please don't even try to). I want to tell you today that if the type of exercise you have been forcing yourself to do feels like torture, then you are totally allowed to stop it! You heard me right. You are *never* required to keep up with the latest trends and put your body through something it hates doing. Will you want to continue with something you don't enjoy long-term? The answer to that is a big fat NO.

Your body is not created to perform the same way as your sister, your best friend, or your spouse. So that being said, you don't have to work out the same way they do if you discover it's not for you. However, as with everything, there is a catch. *You don't have to do a workout you dread, but you DO need to find some form of exercise you enjoy.* Our body thrives when it is kept active! This is a key concept in a healthy lifestyle. So, you can either sign up for every class in your gym or do a variation of YouTube videos from home, or pay for that fitness app, but you DO need to move. Your goal is to keep trying different types of exercise out until you find one that your body likes. You aren't off the hook completely from exercise, but you *never* have to force your body to do something that leaves it feeling awful and worse off than when you started!

Let me take this down to more of a personal level. I myself would rather go skydiving than go for a run. I hate running with a passion and no, I will never "learn to love it." I remember all the way back to middle school when my PE coach wanted us to run the mile. I cared so much about my grades yet I opted out from running it. Instead, I lost points just so I could walk the mile while everyone breezed by me. See, I personally don't get that "runner's high" so many talk about. Instead I get runner's anxiety that makes me feel as if I just chugged a pot of coffee on an empty stomach. I feel shaky and keyed up. It is an awful feeling and therefore I never will force myself to run unless I am literally running for my life. I also recently gave spin class a try and let me tell you, that won't be happening again either.

But what about those flashy headlines we read in fitness magazines that tell us to "push yourself to the max," "cut the excuses," and say there is "no gain without pain"? Listen, I want to really urge you to shut those messages out. Again, our body is not the same as the person next to us. It is not a robot. We are all created unique. I am a firm believer in tuning into your body and doing what makes you feel *good*. Let's refresh on cortisol again for a minute, shall we? If our body is stressed out by having to perform in a way that leaves it feeling like garbage, then we are actually putting our body into fight or flight mode. Basically, our adrenaline is pumping and our cortisol is being secreted by our adrenal glands in heavy doses and then, once again, we find ourselves right back in fat-storage mode.

Have you ever noticed how you can put in hours a week at the gym only to see not even a single pound gone? Well, this typically comes down to two reasons. Either we are not fueling our body properly with whole, real food, or we are stressing our body out to the max by exercising the wrong way. *Our body will tell us what it likes if we will only pay attention!* Some people are made for high-intensity training and feel amazing afterwards. If you are one of them then I honestly envy you! I have always wanted to be able to pop in some earphones and go for a five-mile run on some beautiful trail and be able to have a smile on my face afterwards. I would love to be able enjoy a spin class, but I just really, really don't. After a lot of trial and error I have now found which workouts my body appreciates and benefits the most from. Yoga, Pilates, barre class, and strength training are my go-to's. They keep my body happy, healthy, and fit without causing it excessive stress. I work out on average four to five days a week and I make sure to include rest days as well, as opposed to when I used to work out every single day. I can honestly tell you that now I have a love-love relationship with exercise, but it took years to reach this point.

Over fifty years ago, a man by the name of Dr. Peter D'Adamo came out with the "blood type diet" where he stated his belief that the way we should eat and the way we should exercise is dependent on our blood type. His claim was that people with blood type A, for example, (like me) tend to carry a higher amount of cortisol in their bloodstream than blood type O and therefore they benefit from low-impact exercises such as Pilates, barre, and yoga. Ironically enough, D'Adamo claimed that those with blood type O typically thrive during and after high-intensity training sessions such as running or HIIT workouts. Blood type AB, he believed, benefits from a combination of both.

I personally believe that more studies need to be done on this, but it is an interesting theory to be considered. Regardless of if you choose to believe D'Adamo's theory, I think the point still stands that it is vital for us to tune in to our body during and after a workout. We will only see the results we desire when our body feels that we are really listening and responding to its cues. Only then can our cortisol be managed and kept under control. So keep this in mind the next time you are signing up for a new, trending class at the gym. By all means, feel free to give any new workout a try, but make sure that you are tuning in. I promise that your body will communicate if that workout is for you *if you will only listen.*

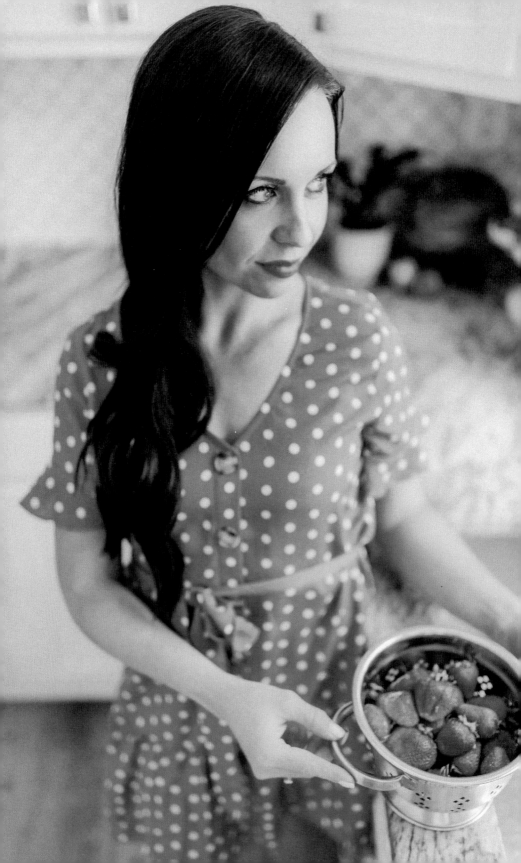

30 Live Healthy With Laura Original Recipes

- Breakfast
  - Blueberry & Avocado Smoothie
  - Cinnamon-Raisin Muffins
  - Spinach & Feta Breakfast Burrito
  - Overnight Chia Seed Pudding
  - Zucchini Muffins
  - Wake-Me-Up Breakfast Smoothie
  - Avocado Toast Three Ways
  - Almond Flour Blueberry Muffins

- Lunch & Dinner
  - Cranberry & Walnut Tuna Salad
  - Broccoli & Salmon Curry Stir-fry
  - Goat Cheese & Sun-dried Tomato Rotini
  - Baked Turkey Meatballs
  - Zucchini Pasta in Garlic Butter
  - Honey-BBQ Chicken Tenderloins
  - Grilled Chicken Salad with Strawberry Vinaigrette
  - Cauliflower Fried Rice
  - Feta, Tomato & Quinoa Salad
  - Broccoli Pesto Farfalle

- Snacks
  - Homemade Hummus Paired with Fresh Veggies
  - Strawberry No-Bake Energy Bars
  - Honey & Cinnamon-Roasted Chickpeas
  - Almond Butter Dip with Apple Slices
  - Crispy Kale Chips
  - Coconut Milk Yogurt & Blueberry Parfait

- Dessert
  - Chocolate-Pecan Brownies
  - Watermelon & Mint Sorbet
  - Cacao & Chia Seed Truffles
  - Crunchy Peanut Butter Cookies
  - Avocado-Chocolate Mousse
  - Coconut-Chocolate Chip Cookies

Breakfast

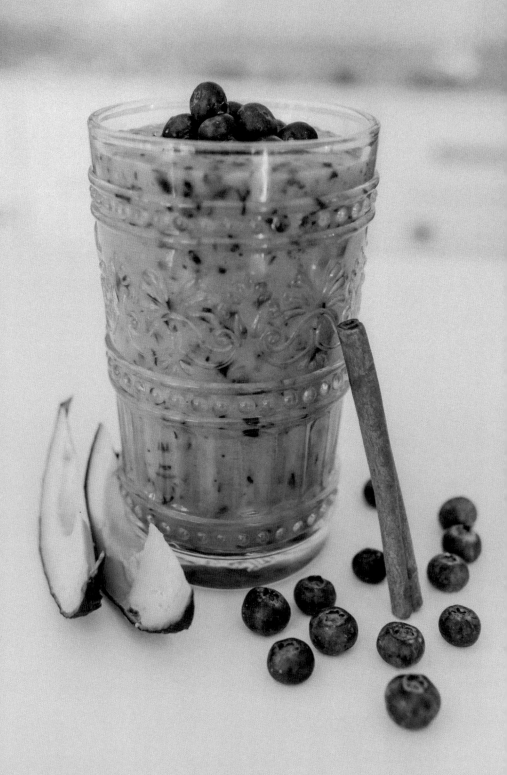

Blueberry & Avocado Smoothie

This smoothie is the perfect combo of healthy fat, natural sugars, fiber, and antioxidants that will give us a little extra pep in our step before we go out the door on those early mornings! It can be whipped together in five minutes or less, and it is kid-friendly! No need to sit down for breakfast if you don't have the time. This smoothie can be carried alongside you all morning long! It will stabilize your blood sugar and get you going after a night of sleep and leave you feeling ready to take on the day!

Ingredients

- 1/2 medium to large, ripe avocado
- 3/4 cup blueberries
- 2 tsp raw honey
- 1 cup organic, unsweetened coconut milk
- 1/4 tsp ground cinnamon
- 1/4 tsp vanilla extract
- 1 cup crushed ice

Directions

In a blender or food processor, add in the crushed ice, cinnamon, vanilla extract, honey, and milk, followed by the avocado and blueberries. Blend well. Serve immediately or stick it in the fridge for later! Enjoy!

*This recipe makes one serving.

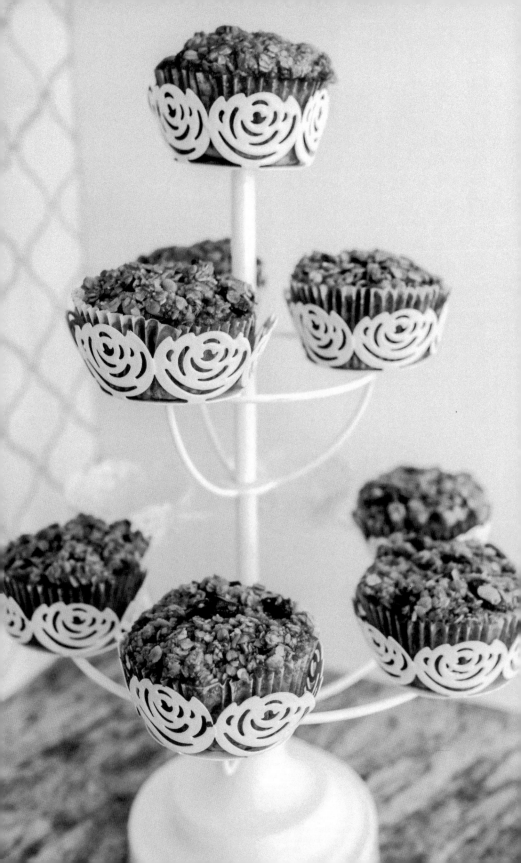

Cinnamon-Raisin Muffins

These muffins are the perfect comfort food on an early morning paired with a cup coffee or as a pick-me-up snack any time of the day! They are easy to transport and are full of energy-packed whole grains, fiber, and protein to keep your digestion in check and your energy steady. Top a muffin with a pat of real butter or coconut oil and trust me, you'll be in heaven! Bake them and freeze half for later, if you would like, and slowly build up your freezer stash for those busy mornings when making breakfast just isn't an option! They can be popped right out of the freezer and be microwaved in 60 seconds and taste just as if they are fresh out of the oven! Try them out. I really think you'll be in love!

Ingredients

- 2 cups quick oats
- 1/3 cup almond flour
- 1/2 cup raisins
- 3 eggs
- 4 tbsp Kerrygold butter (melted)
- 1/2 cup coconut sugar
- 1/2 cup maple syrup
- 1 tsp cinnamon
- 1/2 tsp baking powder

Directions

Preheat your oven to 350°F. Line a muffin tin with 12 paper baking cups. Then, in a medium bowl, add in the oats, almond flour, raisins, coconut sugar, cinnamon, and baking powder and mix well. Then, add in the eggs, melted butter, and syrup and mix thoroughly. Lastly, divide the mixture evenly amongst the muffin tins and bake at 350°F for 20 minutes. Allow the muffins to cool and serve immediately or store in the freezer for later. Enjoy!

*This recipe makes twelve servings.

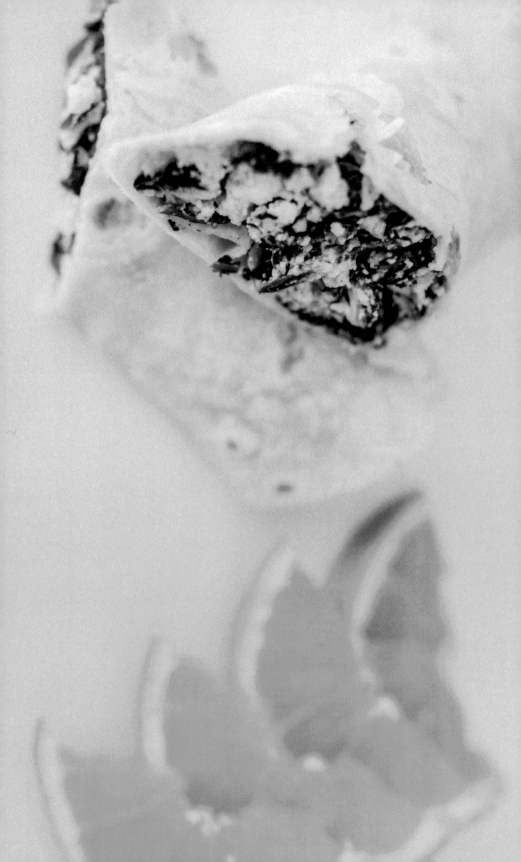

Spinach & Feta Breakfast Burrito

This delicious wrap is my go-to when I am craving something with a little more personality than just my usual scrambled eggs in the morning. It can be thrown together in a pinch and is loaded with greens and amazing, cheesy flavor. It pairs well with any fresh fruit you have on hand and, of course, a cup of coffee. It is so satisfying and filling! I hope you try it and love it as much as I do!

Ingredients

- 1 tbsp coconut oil
- 4 scrambled eggs
- 8 oz feta cheese
- 2 cups fresh baby spinach
- 1/4 tsp ground black pepper
- 4 gluten-free tortillas

Directions

Place a skillet on the stove top, spray it with nonstick spray, and then turn the heat to medium. Then, add in the coconut oil and allow it to melt. Once the oil has melted, add in the baby spinach leaves and sauté them until they have wilted. Add in the eggs, feta, and black pepper and scramble thoroughly. Lay the tortillas flat on separate plates. Divide the egg mixture into four even parts and serve them evenly amongst the tortillas. Wrap the egg mixture tightly in the tortillas and then cut each wrap in half. Serve immediately or freeze for later. Enjoy!

*This recipe makes four servings.

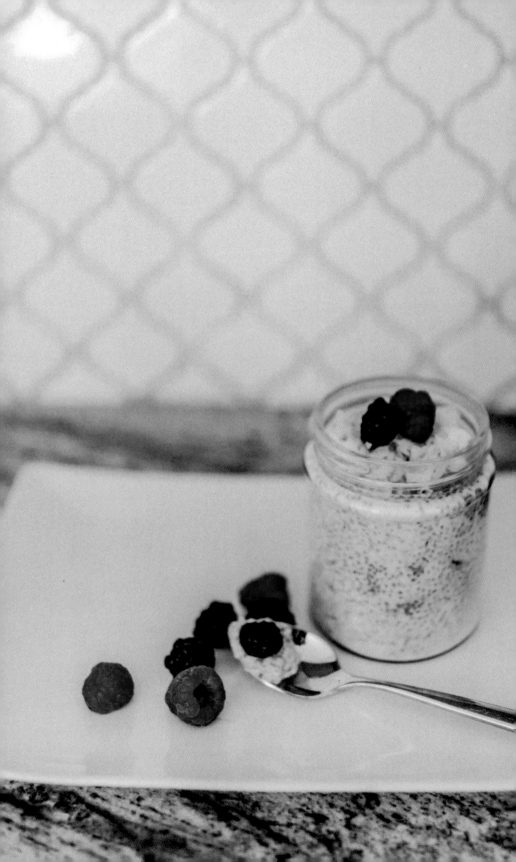

Overnight Chia Seed Pudding

This chia pudding is one of my favorites for those busy days ahead when you know you have to be out the door bright and early the next morning. This can easily be thrown together in a couple of minutes and then stuck in the fridge to set overnight. All you have to do is add the desired toppings in the morning, and you are out the door! Definitely give it a try!

Ingredients

- 4 tbsp chia seeds
- 2/3 cup unsweetened coconut milk
- 2 tsp raw honey
- 1/2 tsp ground cinnamon
- 1/4 tsp vanilla extract
- 1/4 cup fresh berries
- 1 tbsp coconut shavings

Directions

In a small glass or mason jar, mix the ingredients in no specific order and then let sit in the fridge overnight. In the morning, top your pudding with the berries of your choice and coconut shavings and then enjoy!

*This recipe makes one serving.

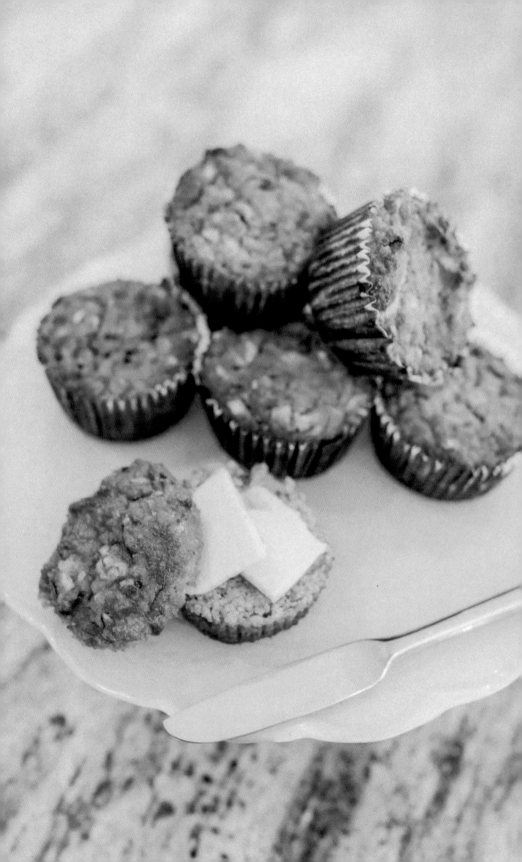

Zucchini Muffins

Are you having trouble getting your kids to eat veggies? Well, then this recipe is for you! Since becoming a mommy, I have found that the best method for getting veggies into my kids is to sneak them in without my children knowing! These muffins are sweet and filling, and the grated zucchini is almost undetectable. You have to try them out!

Ingredients

- 2 cups grated zucchini (about 3 medium zucchini)
- 2 cups almond flour
- 2 eggs
- 2 tbsp melted or liquefied coconut oil
- 1/4 cup raw honey
- 1/4 cup pure maple syrup
- 1/2 cup unsweetened applesauce
- 1/2 tsp vanilla extract
- 2 tsp ground cinnamon
- 1/2 tsp (aluminum-free) baking powder

Directions

Preheat your oven to 350°F. Then, wash and dry your zucchini and cut the ends off. Then, using a cheese grater, grate your zucchini. Pat the grated zucchini dry and set it aside. In a medium bowl, add in the almond flour, cinnamon, and baking powder, followed by the eggs, coconut oil, honey, maple syrup, applesauce, and vanilla extract. Mix well. Lastly, fold in the zucchini. Evenly disperse the muffin mixture in 12 paper muffin cups and bake at 350°F for about 30 minutes or until completely risen. Allow the muffins to cool and either serve right away or store them in the fridge or freezer for later. Enjoy!

*This recipe makes twelve servings.

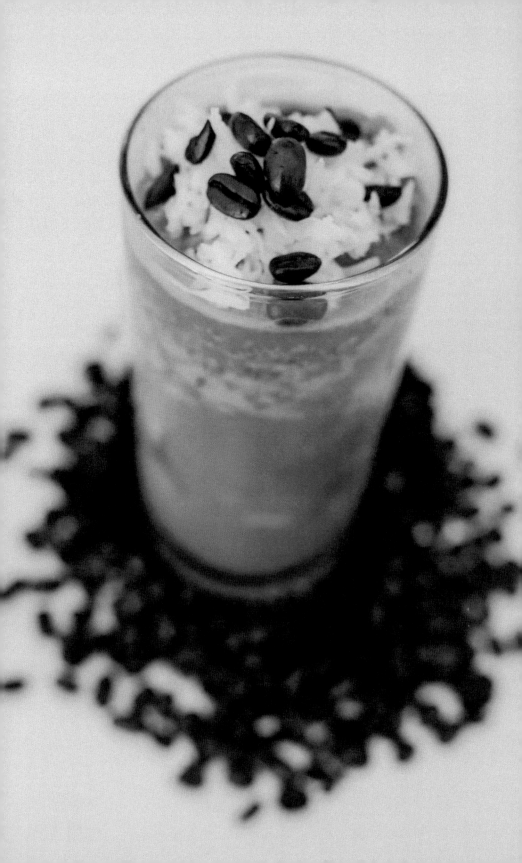

Wake-Me-Up Breakfast Smoothie

Breakfast and coffee all in one? Yes, please! This smoothie has it all! It is the perfect combination of natural caffeine, healthy fats, natural sugar, and protein to get you up and going for the day! I can't even put into words how delicious it is! When I make this, I seriously feel as if I am treating myself with a milkshake for breakfast! It is just that good! This can be thrown together in minutes and taken with you out the door or enjoyed at home. Try it. I know you're going to love it!

Ingredients

- 8 oz brewed, chilled coffee
- 1 diced banana
- 1 tbsp peanut butter
- 1 tbsp pure maple syrup
- 1/2 cup unsweetened coconut milk yogurt
- 1/4 tsp monk fruit
- 1 cup crushed ice

Directions

In a blender, toss in the ice followed by the coffee, peanut butter, maple syrup, yogurt, and monk fruit, followed by the diced banana. Blend until it has reached a smoothie-like texture. Drink immediately, or stick it in the fridge or freezer to chill for later. Enjoy!

*This recipe makes one serving.

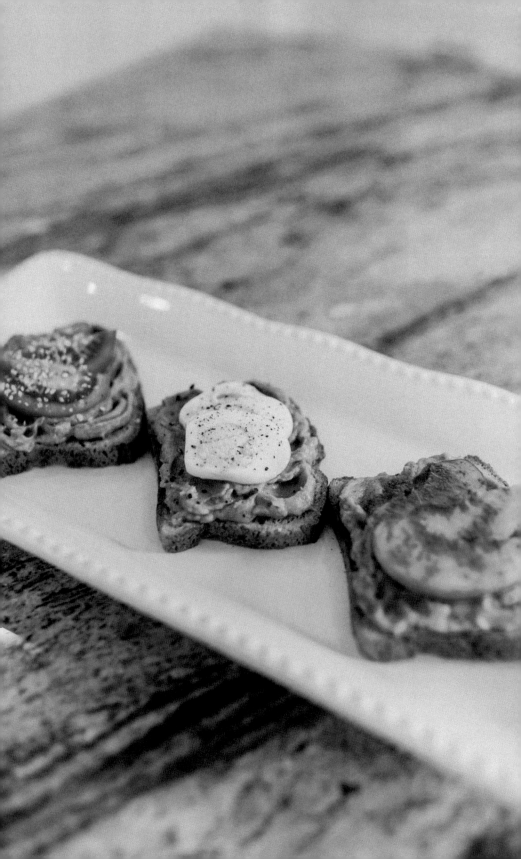

Avocado Toast Three Ways

Creamy avocado smeared on crisp toast. Need I say more? The beauty of avocado toast is it takes on the flavor of whatever you want to top it with. From fruit to various protein sources to veggies and more, you may find yourself surprised to enjoy even seemingly strange combinations! Avocado toast also offers a healthy fat and carbohydrate source to give you some extra pep in your step, and it can be made on even the busiest of mornings! Try out a few of my favorite avocado toast combos, and don't be afraid to branch out and try a few of your own creations as well!

Avocado, Tomato & Everything Seasoning Toast

- 1 piece gluten-free bread (toasted if desired)
- 1/2 smashed avocado
- 1/3 organic tomato
- 2 tsp everything seasoning (I like Amazon's Wholesome Provision brand)

Avocado & Hard-Boiled Egg Toast

- 1 piece gluten-free bread (toasted if desired)
- 1/2 smashed avocado
- 1 sliced, hard-boiled egg
- Salt and pepper to taste

Avocado, Peach & Cinnamon Toast

- 1 piece gluten-free bread (toasted if desired)
- 1/2 smashed avocado
- 1/2 sliced peach
- 1/2 tsp ground cinnamon

Directions

The ingredients speak for themselves! Simply assemble your avocado toast and enjoy!

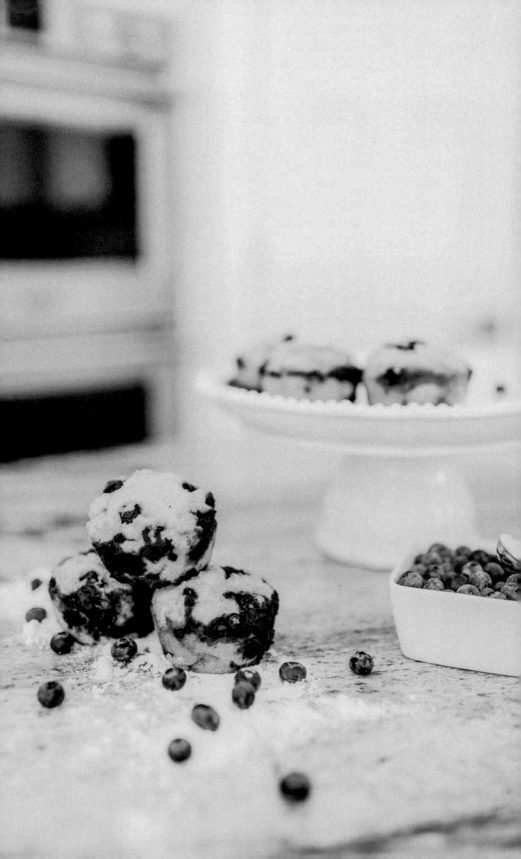

Almond Flour Blueberry Muffins

Who doesn't love the smell of fresh blueberry muffins baking in the kitchen? These muffins are grain-free, but you would never know it! They are loaded with fiber, protein, healthy fat, and antioxidants and are also incredibly filling and juicy! Needless to say, they are a favorite in our household! Make a batch. I can bet you they won't last very long!

Ingredients

- 2 cups almond flour
- 1 cup blueberries
- 3 eggs
- 3 tbsp organic maple syrup
- 1 tsp liquid stevia or monk fruit
- 3 grinds pink Himalayan salt
- ½ cup melted or liquid coconut oil

Directions

Preheat your oven to 350°F. Then, in a medium bowl, mix all of the ingredients together thoroughly (leaving the blueberries for last). Then, carefully fold in the blueberries. Distribute the mixture into an 8-section muffin tin and bake for 15 minutes. Allow the muffins to cool and then serve immediately or store in the fridge or freezer for later. Enjoy!

*This recipe makes eight servings.

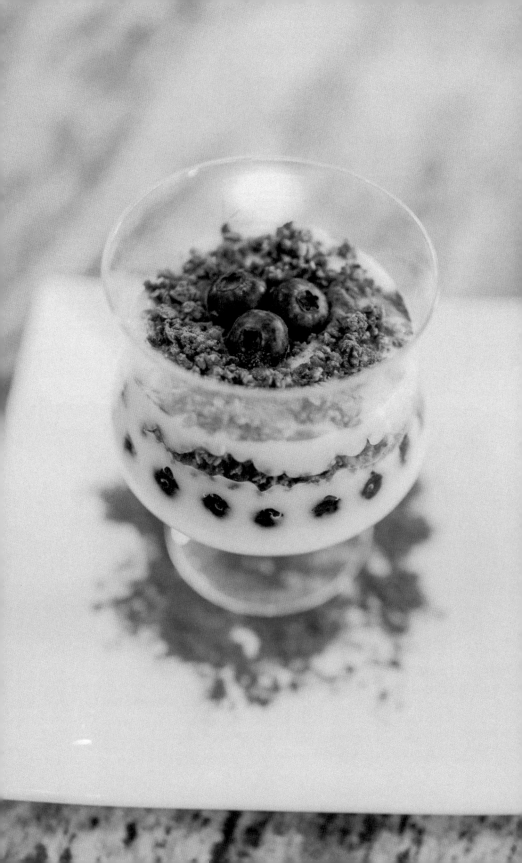

Coconut Milk Yogurt & Blueberry Parfait

This lovely, layered breakfast is a favorite of mine. It can be made in no time when running out the door, and it is one your whole family will love! This layered breakfast is both sweet and creamy, and it has the perfect hint of crunchy texture as well. It also offers protein, healthy fats, and lots of fiber to keep your digestion on point! The assembly process is extremely easy and fun to make too! Try it out!

Parfait Ingredients

- 1/3 cup granola (see recipe)
- 8 oz unsweetened plain or vanilla yogurt (So Delicious is my go-to brand)
- 1/3 cup freshly washed, organic blueberries
- Drizzle of honey

Granola Ingredients

(I recommend making a big batch to have more for later):
- 2 cups quick oats
- 3/4 cup melted or liquid coconut oil
- 3/4 cup honey
- 2 tbsp cinnamon

Directions

Preheat your oven to 350°F. In a medium bowl, combine the quick oats, melted or liquid coconut oil, honey, and cinnamon. Then, using a spatula, evenly spread the mixture on a baking sheet and place in the oven for 20 minutes or until golden brown and then set aside to cool. Once the granola has cooled, use the spatula to break it apart into small chunks. Set aside the appropriate amount for your parfait and then store the rest in a Ziploc bag in a cool, dry place. Then, in a small trifle glass, start assembling your parfait. Start with a layer of yogurt, then a layer of blueberries, then a layer of granola, and repeat till you reach the top of your glass. For an extra sweet kick, add a drizzle of honey and then enjoy!

This recipe makes one serving.

Lunch and Dinner Recipes

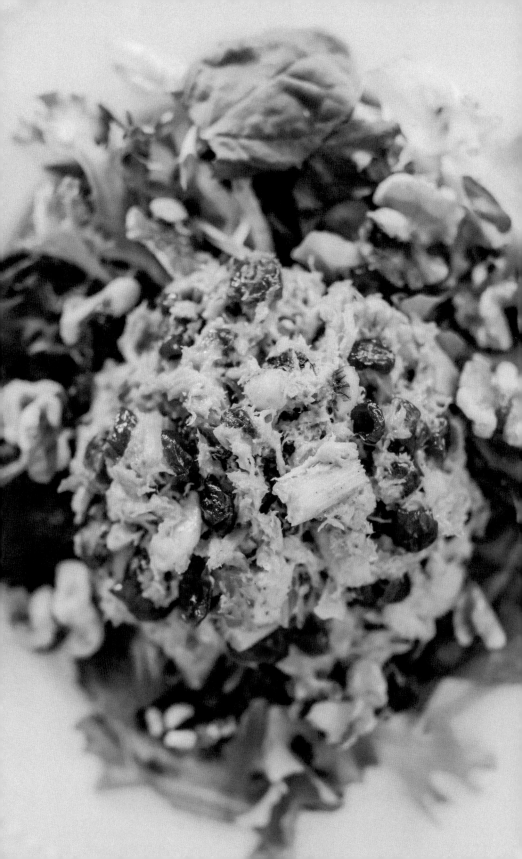

Cranberry & Walnut Tuna Salad

This tuna salad is one of my favorite quick and easy lunches or dinners for those days when extra time cooking in the kitchen just isn't an option. This salad requires minimal effort, but it offers a punch of protein, healthy fats, fiber, and a sweet kick as well! Make it into a sandwich, eat it on gluten-free crackers, or eat it straight out of the bowl. Either way, I know you are going to love it!

Ingredients

- 4 packets or cans of tuna (in water)
- 6 tbsp real mayonnaise
- 2 tsp curry powder
- 2/3 cup dried cranberries
- 2/3 cup diced celery
- 8 cups field greens

Directions

Simply toss all of the ingredients in a bowl in no specific order and mix well. Serve immediately over field greens or store for up to three days. Enjoy!

*This recipe makes two servings.

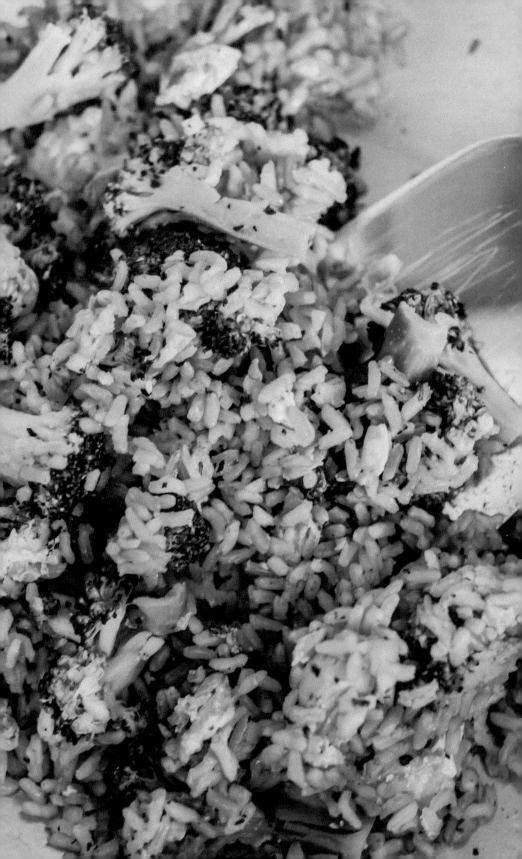

Broccoli & Salmon Curry Stir-fry

Who doesn't love a 10-minute meal full of protein, healthy fats, whole grains, and veggies all in one? This stir-fry is full of flavor and is perfect for those who enjoy both Thai or Indian cuisine and those who are fans of seafood! If you make the rice ahead of time (I make mine in the Instant Pot), then you can have a balanced, home-cooked meal in no time! Try it out!

Ingredients

- 4 cups cooked brown rice (about 11/2 cup dried)
- 16 oz or four small fillets wild Alaskan salmon (skin off)
- 4 tbsp EVOO (extra virgin olive oil)
- 4 cups broccoli
- 2 tsp curry powder
- 2 tsp pink Himalayan salt
- 1 tsp garlic powder
- 1 tsp dried basil

Directions

Spray a medium-sized skillet with nonstick spray and then turn the heat on your stove top to medium. Then, add in the salmon and cook thoroughly. Dice it up in the pan into bite-sized pieces. Then, toss in the broccoli, rice, and seasonings and sauté it all together. Serve the stir-fry immediately off the stove and enjoy!

*This recipe makes four servings.

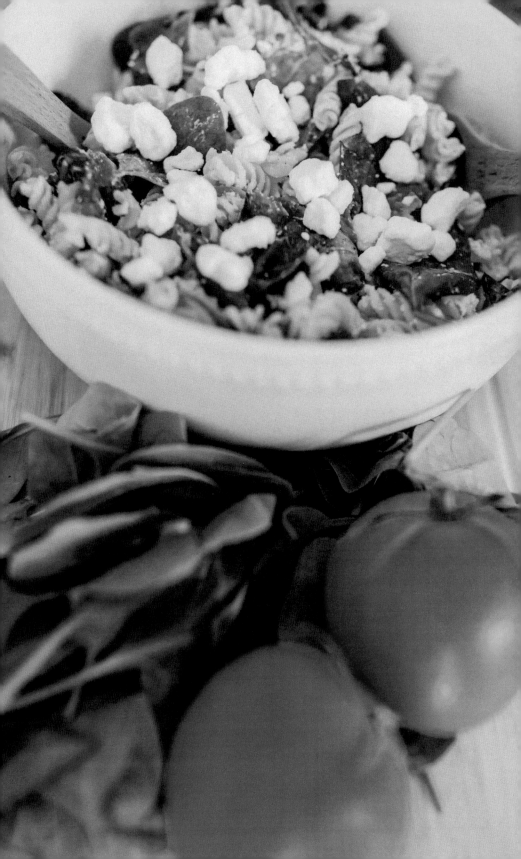

Goat Cheese & Sun-dried Tomato Rotini

I can't even express how much pasta makes me smile. I love Italian food, and I love a delicious, homemade comfort meal that leaves me feeling amazing and not bogged down. This gluten-free pasta dish is a great source of whole grains, protein, calcium, iron, fiber, and veggies! It can be eaten immediately or made in bulk and refrigerated for the week ahead or even frozen for later! Give it a try!

Ingredients

- 16 oz gluten-free, dried rotini pasta
- 8 oz crumbled goat cheese
- 1 1/3 cup unseasoned, sun-dried tomatoes
- 2 cups fresh baby spinach leaves
- 2 tbsp EVOO (extra virgin olive oil)
- 1/2 tsp pink Himalayan salt
- 1/4 tsp black pepper

Directions

Boil your pasta according to the package's directions. Then, drain your noodles and add them back into the pot. Add the olive oil, toss in the spinach leaves, and mix well on low heat until they are wilted. Then, add the tomatoes, goat cheese, salt, and pepper and continue to stir on low until the cheese is completely melted and dispersed throughout the pasta. Serve immediately or store in the fridge or freezer for later. Enjoy!

This recipe makes four servings.

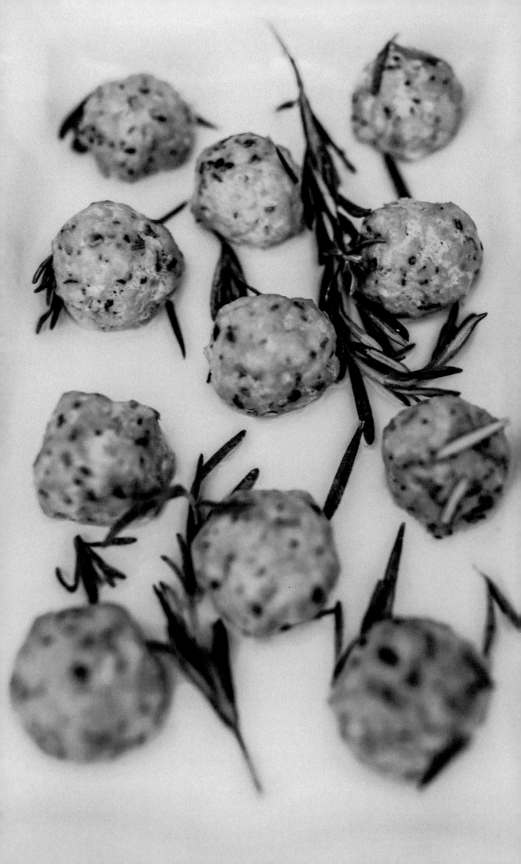

Baked Turkey Meatballs

It is no secret that I am all about convenience and simplicity. These meatballs are perfect for even the busiest of weeknights! They make great leftovers for the next day's lunch, and they also freeze well for later. They can be mixed up, rolled into balls, and thrown in the oven in no time! They are loaded with lean protein and loads of natural flavors. Trust me, their taste will not disappoint! They can be added to your favorite pasta dish or paired with a fresh salad or some steamed veggies. I hope you give them a try and discover how simple a healthy, home-cooked meal can be to make even when you are short on time!

Ingredients

- 1 lb ground turkey
- 2 tsp Italian seasoning
- 1 tsp garlic powder
- 1 tsp crushed and dried rosemary
- 1 tsp pink Himalayan salt
- 2 tbsp EVOO (extra virgin olive oil)

Directions

In a medium-sized bowl, add in the ground turkey followed by the olive oil and the seasoning and herbs on top. Then, using your hands, mix the seasonings well into the ground turkey and roll the turkey mixture into about 12 one-inch balls. Stick the meatballs one inch apart on a Pyrex dish sprayed with nonstick spray and bake at 375°F for 25 minutes. Eat immediately or freeze for later. Enjoy!

This recipe makes four servings.

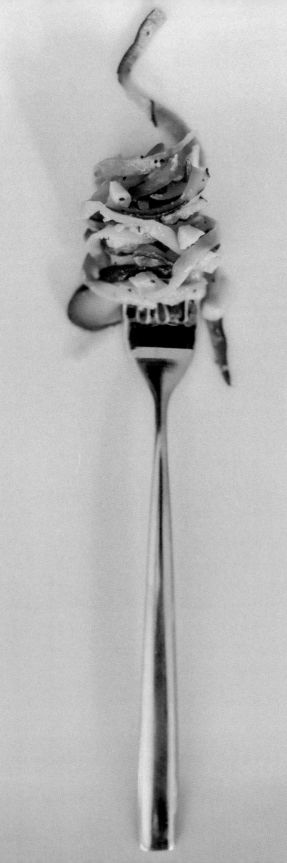

Zucchini Pasta in Garlic Butter

"Zoodles" have always been my go-to when I am in the mood for a quick meal that is filling yet still light at the same time. This delicious dish is loaded with flavor, immunity-boosting antioxidants, and healthy fats. It can be thrown together in minutes and eaten on its own or topped with your protein of choice. I personally love them topped with my Baked Turkey Meatballs! Branch out and try them. You won't be sorry!

Ingredients

- 4 large, spiraled zucchini
- 4 tbsp real butter
- 1/2 tsp black pepper
- 1/2 tsp pink Himalayan salt
- 6 minced garlic cloves (fresh and not from a jar)
- 1/2 cup grated parmesan cheese to garnish (optional)

Directions

Add the butter to a large skillet and turn the heat on the stove top to medium. Once the butter is melted, add in the minced garlic and sauté for five minutes and then toss in the zucchini, followed by the remaining spices. Allow the zucchini to cook down and sauté for a remaining 1-2 minutes. Add parmesan cheese or another protein of choice on top, if desired, and then serve immediately. Enjoy!

*This recipe makes four servings.

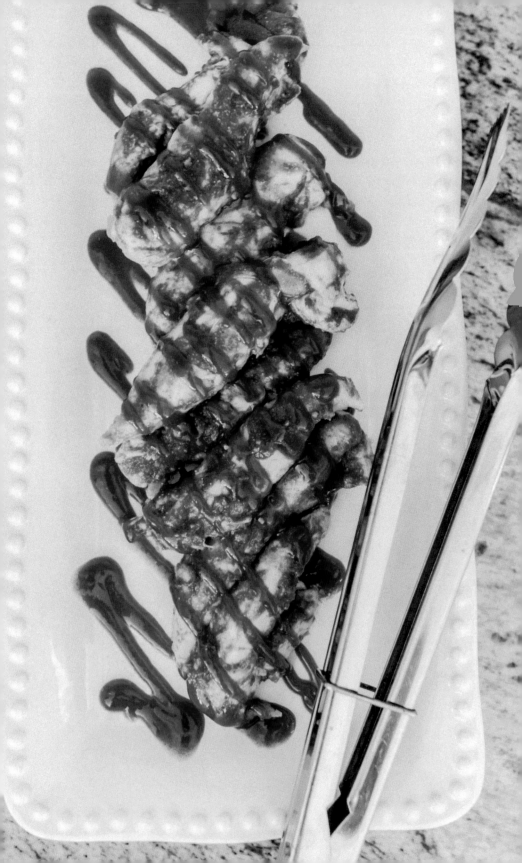

Honey-BBQ Chicken Tenderloins

Barbecue is so incredibly delicious and has always been a favorite of mine, especially in the warmer months! Unfortunately, though, most store-bought brands are packed with refined sugar or high-fructose corn syrup, so I decided to create my own. This sauce offers all of the flavors of traditional honey-barbecue sauce but with clean, good-for-you ingredients! Make a large batch and store it in the fridge for whenever you may need it. It is delicious on nearly any meat or fish. Whip some up and give it a try!

Ingredients

- 2 lbs boneless, skinless chicken tenderloins

BBQ Sauce
- 4 tbsp ketchup (high-fructose corn-syrup-free)
- 1 tbsp honey
- 1 tbsp apple cider vinegar
- 1/2 tsp garlic powder
- 1/2 tsp paprika
- 1/2 tsp pink Himalayan salt
- 1 tsp Worcestershire sauce

Directions

In a small bowl, mix the ketchup, honey, garlic powder, paprika, and salt together. Then, add in the apple cider vinegar and Worcestershire sauce and mix again. Once the sauce is completely mixed together, rub an even, thin layer of the sauce over raw, skinless chicken tenderloins and bake in the oven at 350°F for 30 minutes or stick them on the grill if preferred. Pair the cooked chicken with steamed broccoli (one cup per person) and enjoy!

I highly suggest you quadruple this sauce recipe and save some in the fridge for later.

This recipe makes four servings.

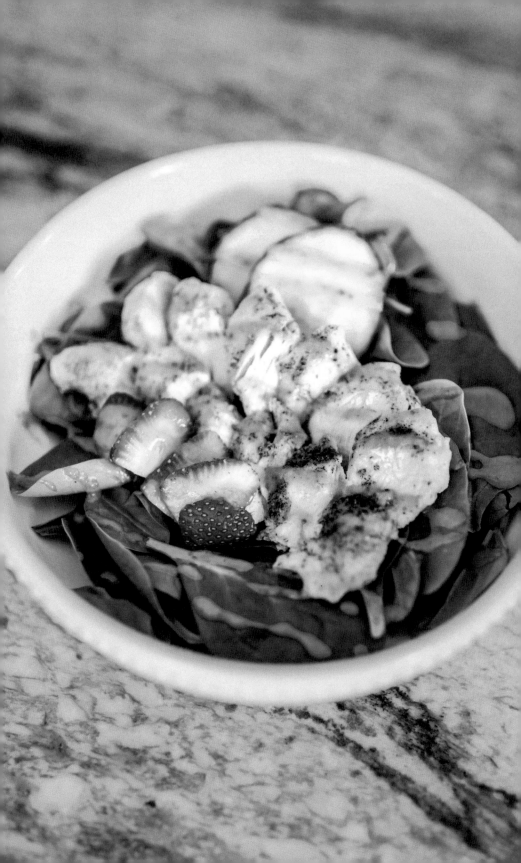

Grilled Chicken Salad with Strawberry Vinaigrette

Grilled chicken salads tend to carry quite a boring reputation these days. However, if you do it right and jazz salads up, they really can be out-of-this-world amazing! I find this salad so refreshing and filling. It offers all of the greens, healthy fats, and tangy strawberry flavor to keep your taste buds hooked. Try it out next time you are in the mood for a delicious, energizing meal that can be made in 10 minutes or less!

Ingredients

- 1 lb grilled or sautéed sliced chicken breast
- 4 cups field greens
- 1 medium cucumber
- 1 cup diced strawberries
- 1/2 cup diced walnuts
- 1/2 cup feta cheese (optional)

Strawberry Vinaigrette

- 6 medium strawberries
- 2 tbsp extra virgin olive oil
- 2 tbsp apple cider vinegar
- 1 pinch or 1/8 tsp pink Himalayan salt
- 1 tbsp lemon juice
- 1 tsp honey

Directions

Cook your chicken breast however you desire and slice thinly. Then, in a food processor or a blender, blend up the ingredients for the strawberry vinaigrette. Once the dressing has reached a smooth, creamy texture, start to assemble the salad. Start by first adding in the greens, then the cucumber, strawberries, feta cheese (if desired), and then the walnuts. Lastly, drizzle the dressing evenly over the salad and enjoy!

This recipe makes two servings.

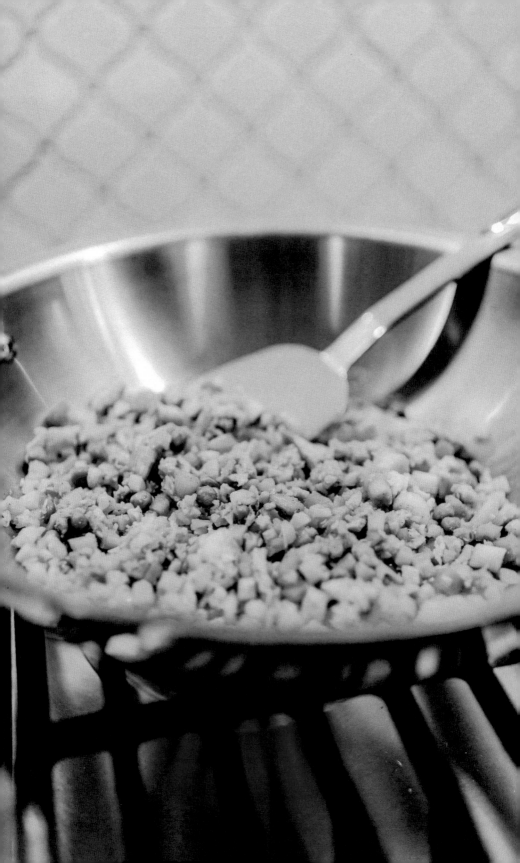

Cauliflower Fried Rice

Fried rice ... need I really say more? It is a favorite of mine whether I am eating hibachi, Chinese, or Thai food. I created this lighter version, loaded with veggies and fiber and protein, to provide all the flavors of traditional fried rice yet without the heaviness. It is such a filling dish that it can be eaten on its own or paired with your protein of choice. I hope you give it a try and find it as tasty as I do!

Ingredients

- 12 oz riced cauliflower
- 1/3 cup chopped green onions
- 3/4 cup frozen peas and carrots (thawed)
- 3 eggs (scrambled)
- 2 tbsp pure sesame oil
- 2 tbsp coconut aminos
- 1 tbsp minced garlic
- 1/4 tsp black pepper

Directions

In a medium skillet or wok, add in the sesame oil and minced garlic and sauté for 2-3 minutes. Then, add the riced cauliflower, onions, peas, carrots, and scrambled eggs all together and stir well. Drizzle the coconut aminos on top and stir until evenly distributed throughout. Lastly, top the dish with the black pepper and enjoy!

*This recipe makes two servings.

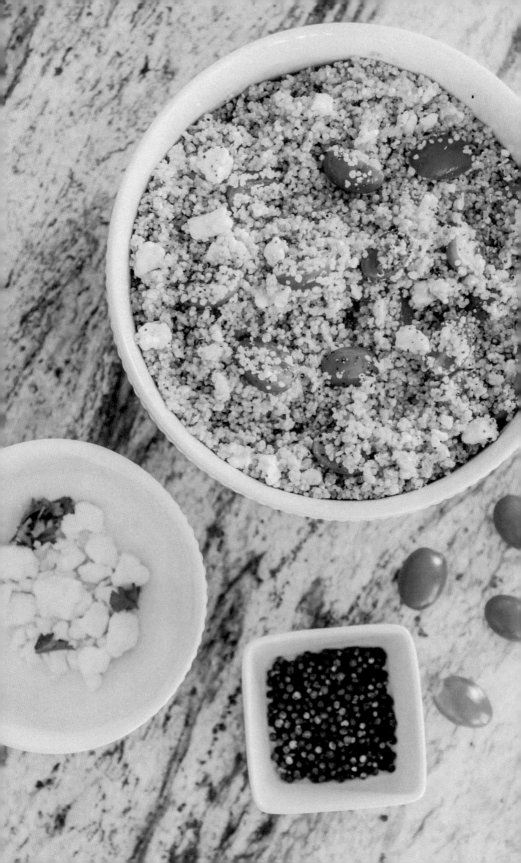

Feta, Tomato & Quinoa Salad

This grain bowl is one of my favorite creations. It is so energizing, and is made up of a delicious combination of salty feta and sweet, juicy tomatoes, tossed in one of the most protein-rich grains there is, then bathed in heart-healthy, antioxidant-rich olive oil. It is the ultimate Mediterranean dish, and it is incredibly simple to make! It stores well in the fridge for days and is a great crowd-pleaser as well! Check it out!

Ingredients

- 1 cup dried quinoa
- 8 oz crumbled feta cheese
- 4 tbsp extra virgin olive oil (EVOO)
- 1 cup organic cherry tomatoes (cut in half)
- Black pepper

Directions

Cook the quinoa according to the package directions and allow it to cool in the refrigerator or at room temperature for a few minutes. Then, once cooled, add in the halved cherry tomatoes, feta cheese, and olive oil and toss thoroughly. Lastly, top the dish with ground black pepper and enjoy!

This recipe makes two servings.

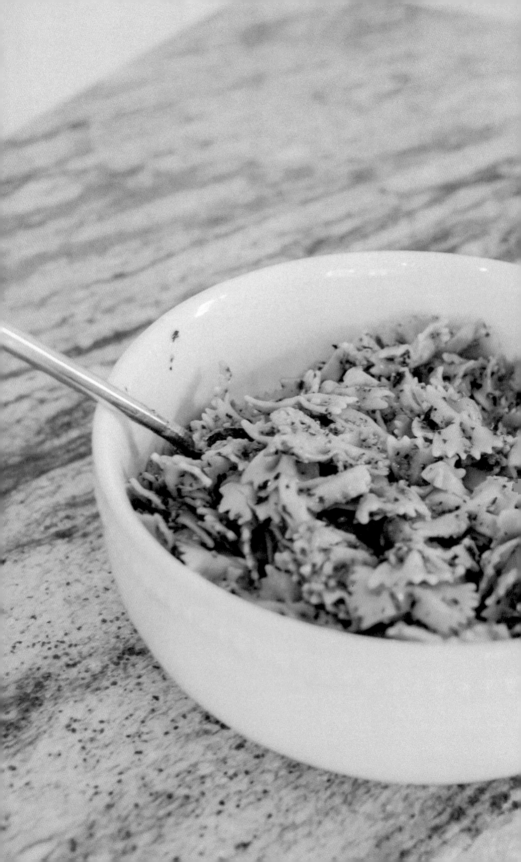

Broccoli Pesto Farfalle

Italian food will always be my favorite comfort cuisine of choice. This pesto, specifically, is one of my favorites! It is loaded with one of my favorite herbs (basil) and has just enough immunity-boosting garlic to give it a kick of flavor! It is a creamy sauce whether or not you choose to include the parmesan cheese or choose to leave it out and make it vegan style. Whichever way you try it, you won't be disappointed!

Ingredients

- 1 cup steamed broccoli
- 1/2 oz fresh basil
- 2 cloves garlic
- 3 tbsp extra virgin olive oil (EVOO)
- 4 oz shredded parmesan cheese (**optional if you prefer vegan style**)
- 12 oz gluten-free farfalle

Directions

Boil the pasta according to the box's directions. Then, in a food processor, add in the basil, garlic, steamed broccoli, olive oil, and parmesan cheese (if desired). Then, pulse until it has reached a creamy, sauce-like consistency. Drain the pasta and then thoroughly mix in the pesto, and you are ready to eat! Enjoy!

*This recipe makes four servings.

Snacks

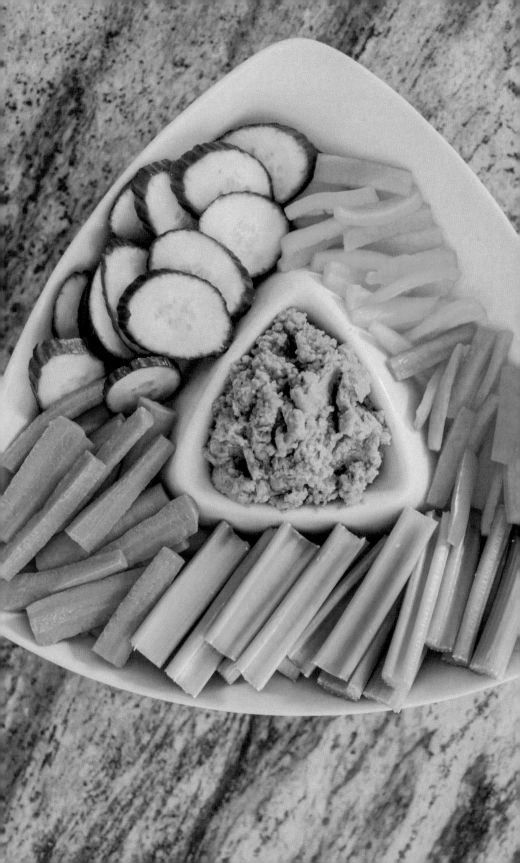

Homemade Hummus Paired With Fresh Veggies

Creamy hummus is always my go-to plant-based snack of choice! I love the texture of pureed chickpeas with a hint of spice on crisp, cool veggies, or gluten-free crackers. This hummus recipe is extremely simple to make, and it can also be made ahead of time in bulk and stored for days in the fridge. Eat it at home or on the go! Either way, I am sure you are going to love it!

Ingredients

- 15 oz can chickpeas
- 3 tbsp extra virgin olive oil
- 1/8 tsp paprika
- 1/4 tsp cumin
- 1/4 tsp curry
- 1/2 tsp garlic powder
- 1/8 tsp or one pinch of pink Himalayan salt
- Fresh-cut veggies of choice

Directions

In a food processor, add in the chickpeas, extra virgin olive oil, spices, and puree until creamy. Then, serve immediately at room temperature or chill in the fridge for later.

This recipe makes two servings.

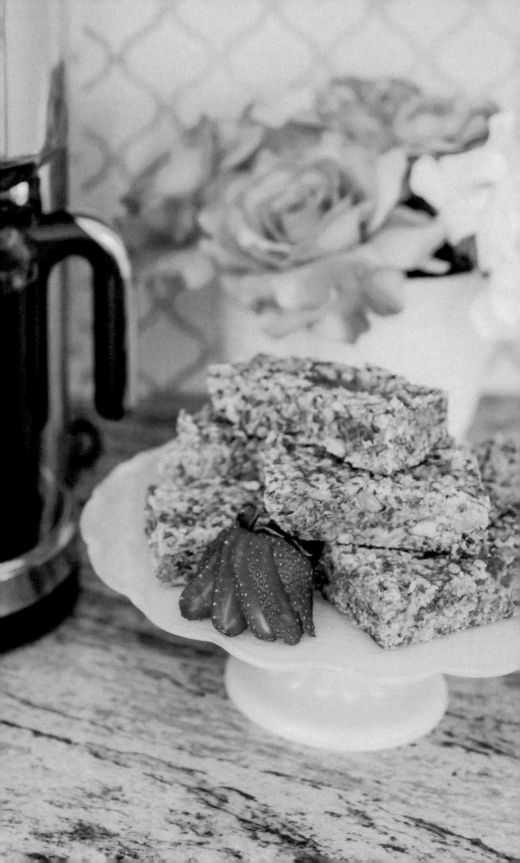

Strawberry No-Bake Energy Bars

If you are a granola and strawberry fan, then these bars are for you! They are chewy and packed with fiber, protein, omegas, and natural sugars! They are perfect as a snack on the go, and they are also kid-friendly. Make a batch and enjoy these as a sweet and energizing pick-me-up at any time of the day!

Ingredients

- 2 cups quick oats
- 1/2 cup raw honey
- 3/4 cup melted almond butter
- 1/2 cup chopped almonds
- 1 cup chopped strawberries
- 1/4 cup flax seeds
- 1/4 cup melted coconut oil
- 1/2 tsp ground cinnamon

Directions

In a medium bowl, mix the ingredients together, starting with the dry ingredients first and leaving the wet ingredients for last. Then, line an 8 × 8 Pyrex dish with parchment paper and pour the mixture into the dish. Stick the dish in the refrigerator to harden for two hours. Remove the dish from the fridge and carefully pull up the edges of the parchment paper and remove the bars. Lay the bars on a baking sheet or a clean countertop and cut evenly into 8 rectangular pieces. Wrap each bar individually in plastic or place each one in a Ziploc bag and then enjoy one immediately or place the bars back in the refrigerator for later. Enjoy!

*This recipe makes eight servings.

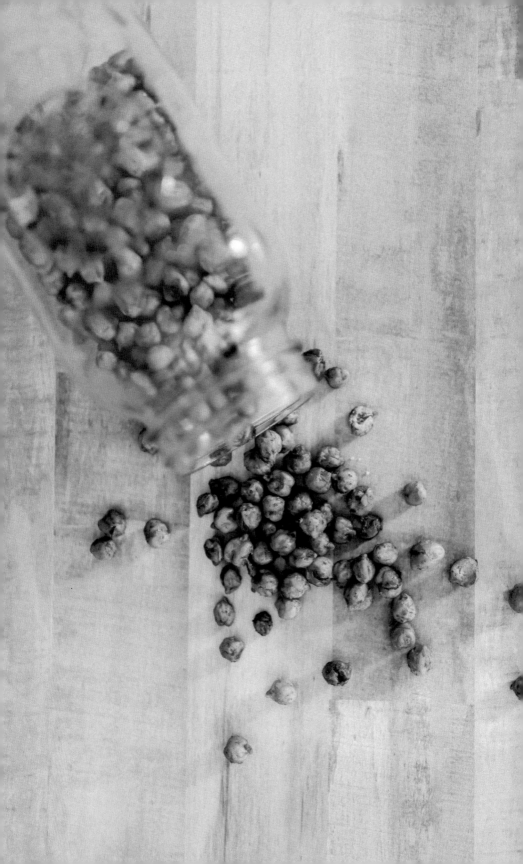

Honey & Cinnamon-Roasted Chickpeas

These crunchy and sweet little legumes make the perfect snack and treat! This recipe is loaded with protein, healthy fats, fiber, B vitamins, and more! They are the perfect way to take care of your sweet tooth and balance your blood sugar at the same time. They take only a few minutes to make, and they smell up your kitchen in the process! Roast some up and try them for yourself!

Ingredients

- 25 oz can chickpeas
- 1/4 cup honey
- 1/4 cup coconut sugar
- 1 tbsp cinnamon

Directions

Preheat your oven to 400°F. Then, open and drain the can of chickpeas and place them on a sprayed baking sheet and pat them dry with a paper towel. Bake the plain chickpeas at 400°F for 15 minutes. Then, in a small mixing bowl, add in the roasted chickpeas, honey, coconut sugar, and cinnamon and toss thoroughly. Pour the chickpeas on the pan and disperse evenly. Bake them for 15 more minutes. Allow them to cool and then start snacking on them immediately or store at room temperature for later. Enjoy!

*This recipe makes two servings.

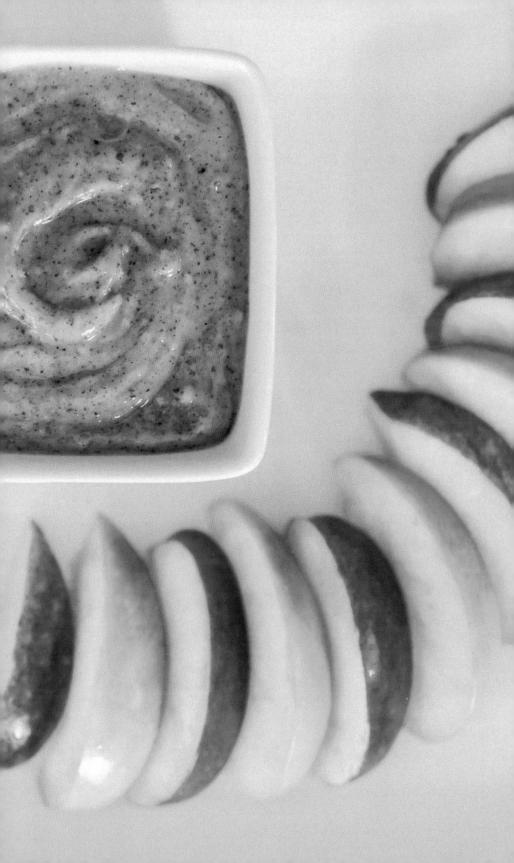

Almond Butter Fruit Dip

Creamy, sweet almond butter dip with crisp, fresh fruit is my kind of snack! This dairy-free and sugar-free dip provides the perfect combination of both nutty flavor and sweet honey. I really struggle to get enough of this delicious dip, and my kids are big fans of it too! It can be made in a flash, and it can last in the fridge for days or be served right away. Give it a try!

Ingredients

- 1/2 cup coconut milk yogurt
- 3 tbsp almond butter
- 1 tbsp honey
- 1/2 tsp ground cinnamon
- 1 pinch or 1/8 tsp pink Himalayan salt
- 1/4 tsp vanilla extract

Directions

In a small bowl, mix the above ingredients together thoroughly and then serve with fresh-cut fruit of your choice. Enjoy!

This recipe makes one serving.

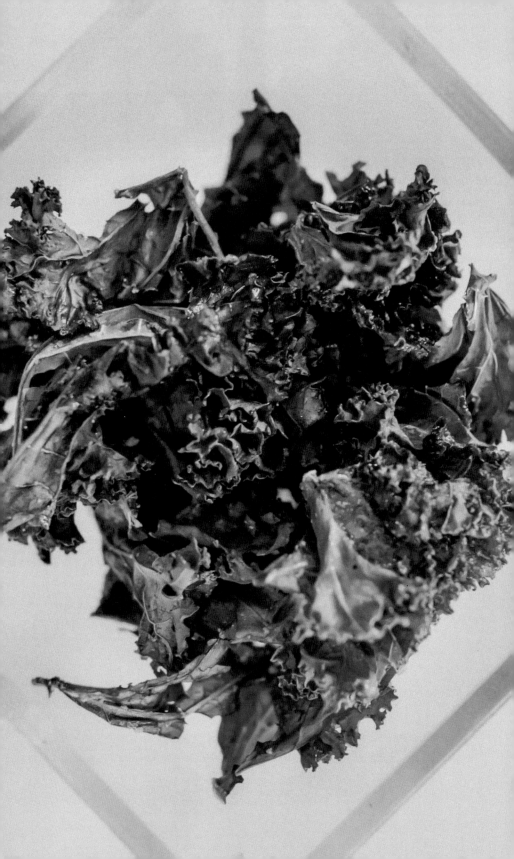

Crispy Kale Chips

Who doesn't love a crunchy, nutritious snack that is packed with vitamins, healthy fats, and antioxidants and also loaded with flavor? These kale chips can be made in bulk and enjoyed by you and your family all week long! Trust me, they won't disappoint. Try them out!

Ingredients

- 4 cups kale (stalks removed)
- 3 tbsp extra virgin olive oil
- 2 tsp nutritional yeast
- 1 tsp garlic powder
- 1/8 tsp pink Himalayan salt

Directions

Preheat your oven to 325°F. Spread the kale leaves evenly on a large baking sheet (sprayed first with nonstick spray) and evenly drizzle with the olive oil, followed by an even sprinkle of both the nutritional yeast and garlic powder. Stick the seasoned kale leaves in the oven on the middle rack for 15 minutes or until crispy. Allow the kale chips to cool and then enjoy right away or store them in a sealed container at room temperature for later! Enjoy!

This recipe makes two servings.

Dessert

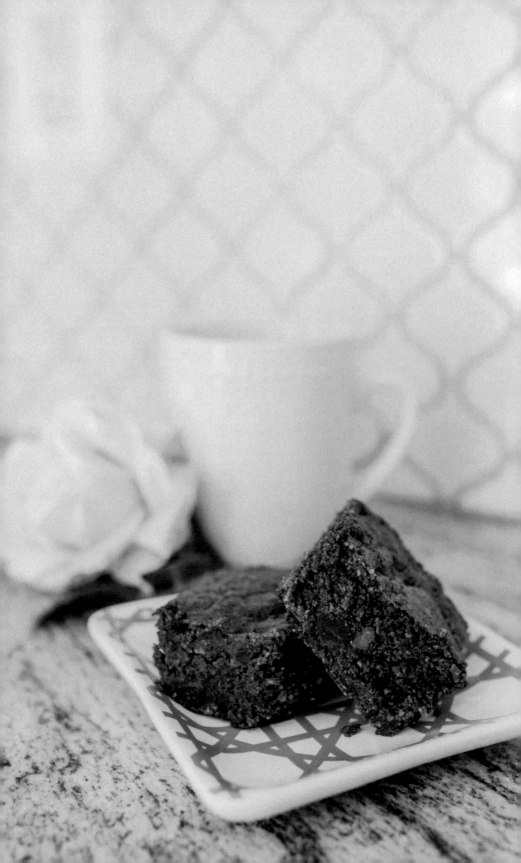

Chocolate-Pecan Brownies

I really can't put into words how decadent this brownie recipe is. If you are a chocolate lover like I am, then you need to have these brownies in your life! They are rich and moist and loaded with lots of antioxidant-rich cacao, gluten-free and protein-rich almond flour, and a chocolate flavor that's to die for! Make a batch and you will see what I am raving about!

Ingredients

- 1/2 cup rice flour
- 1 1/2 cup almond flour
- 1/2 cup Enjoy Life dark chocolate chips
- 1/4 cup Enjoy Life dark chocolate chips (set aside for later)
- 3/4 cup coconut oil
- 2 tbsp cocoa powder
- 3/4 cup organic maple syrup
- 1/2 cup coconut sugar
- 1/2 tsp baking powder
- 2 eggs
- 3/4 cup chopped pecans
- 1/4 cup coconut milk

Directions

Preheat your oven to 375°F. Then, in a small saucepan, cook together the 1/2-cup chocolate chips and the coconut oil on low heat until melted. In the meantime, grab a medium bowl and add in all of the dry ingredients (aside from the remainder of the chocolate chips) and then stir. Then, add in the maple syrup, eggs, coconut milk, and melted chocolate sauce. Once the batter is combined well, add in the remaining chocolate chips and stir well. Pour the batter mixture into an 8 × 8 baking pan that's been sprayed with nonstick spray. Place the brownies in the oven and allow them to bake for 30 minutes. Allow them to cool on the stove top and then enjoy!

*This recipe makes eight brownies.

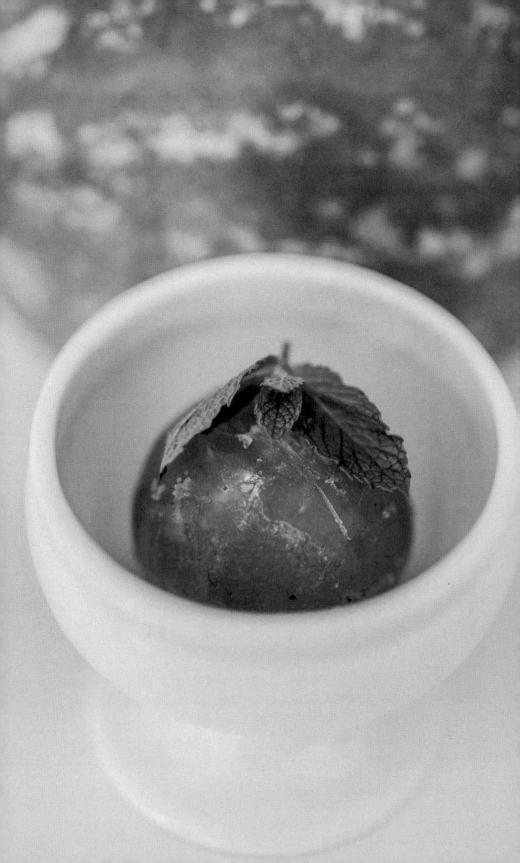

Watermelon & Mint Sorbet

I love this refreshing, icy treat! It is perfect for those hot summer days, but it can totally be enjoyed any time of the year! I personally love it as a palate cleanser after a savory meal, and my kids love it as an afternoon treat! It is loaded with antioxidants as well as lemon and mint to help aid digestion. Give it a try! You will love it!

Ingredients

- 4 cups diced, seedless watermelon
- 3 tbsp fresh-squeezed lemon juice
- 2 tsp liquid monk fruit extract
- 1 oz or 10 fresh mint leaves, finely chopped

Directions

In a blender, add in the lemon juice, monk fruit, and mint leaves, leaving the watermelon for last. Then, blend until you have reached a smoothie-like texture and pour into silicone molds or into a Pyrex dish to freeze overnight (or at least 8 hours). Lastly, pop the molds into a dish or scoop the sorbet out and enjoy!

*This recipe makes four servings.

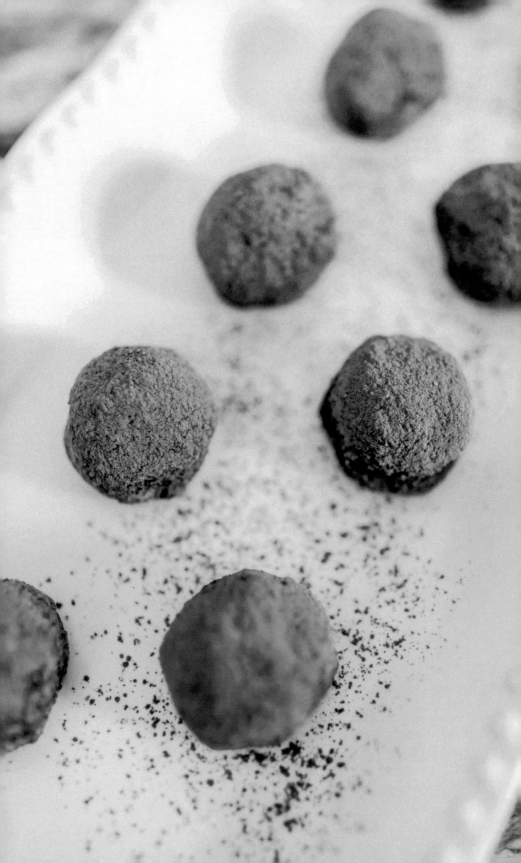

Cacao & Chia Seed Truffles

I couldn't resist sharing yet another chocolate lover's treat. These chocolate truffles with a brownie-like texture are loaded with protein, fiber, and omegas and are the perfect sweet pick-me-up any time of the day! They can stay fresh in the fridge for days, and they are popular with the kids as well! Try them out!

Ingredients

- 2 cups almond flour
- 1/2 cup coconut sugar
- 1/4 cup chia seeds
- 1/4 cup maple syrup
- 2 tbsp cacao powder
- 2 tsp ground cinnamon
- 2 tbsp cacao powder (set aside for later)
- 1/4 cup coconut milk

Directions

In a medium bowl, add in the almond flour, coconut sugar, chia seeds, cacao powder, and cinnamon and mix well. Pour in the maple syrup and coconut milk and mix again. Then, in a smaller bowl, add the 2 tbsp cacao powder and set aside. Wash and dry your hands. Roll one-inch balls by hand, toss them around in the cacao powder, and set them on a plate sprayed with nonstick spray. Once finished, stick the truffles in the fridge to chill for at least one hour before serving. Enjoy!

This recipe makes about twenty-four truffles.

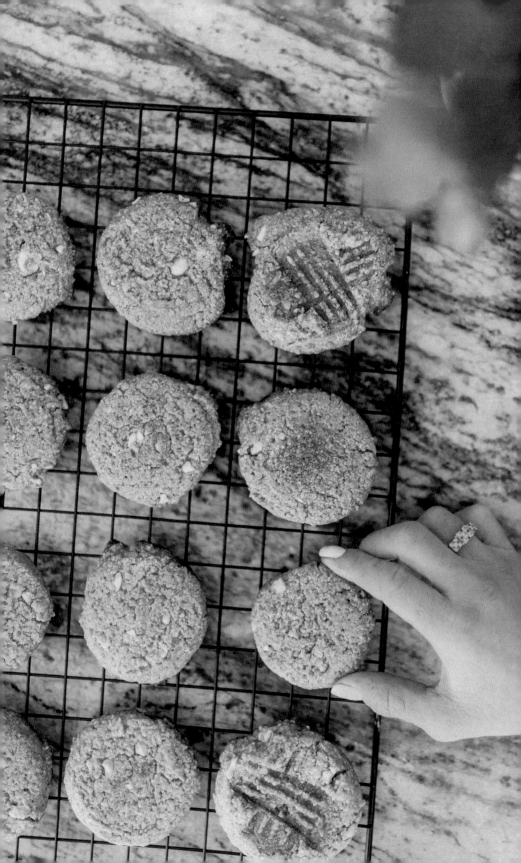

Crunchy Peanut Butter Cookies

As much as I love chocolate, I am equally a fan of anything peanut butter! I love its creamy, nutty flavor. Now, sweeten it up with a little coconut sugar and turn it into a cookie, and then we are really talking! These cookies are loaded with protein, healthy fats, and fiber! They are the perfect, good-for-you sweet treat that will leave you energized and satisfied! Give them a try!

Ingredients

- 2 cups almond flour
- 1/3 cup rice flour
- 1/2 cup coconut sugar
- 1/4 cup honey
- 1 tsp baking powder
- 1/2 cup melted coconut oil
- 1/2 cup chopped peanuts
- 1/2 cup softened peanut butter
- 2 eggs

Directions

Preheat your oven to 350°F. Then, in a medium bowl, combine the almond flour, rice flour, coconut sugar, baking powder, and chopped peanuts. Then, soften the peanut butter and coconut oil in the microwave for 30 seconds each and add it in along with the honey and eggs and mix well. Then, using a two-tablespoon cookie scoop, portion out your cookie dough and place on a baking sheet sprayed with nonstick spray, leaving a one-inch gap in between. Allow the cookies to bake for 15 minutes and let them cool before storing or serving. Enjoy!

This recipe makes twelve cookies.

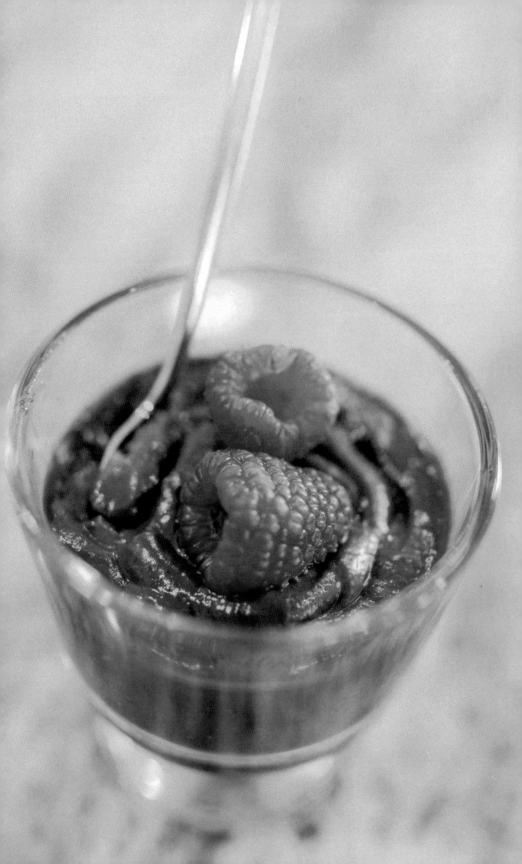

Avocado-Chocolate Mousse

This mousse is the ultimate chocolate indulgence. It is my own spin off of chocolate pudding, and it is loaded with healthy fats, antioxidants, and it is also sugar-free! It takes less than 5 minutes to whip up and can be stored in the fridge for days! Try it out!

Ingredients

- 3 large to medium (or 4 small) ripe avocados
- 3 ripe bananas
- 2 tsp organic ground cinnamon
- 4 tbsp organic cacao powder
- 1 tsp liquid monk fruit or stevia
- 1/3 cup organic, unsweetened coconut milk

Directions

In a food processor or blender, add in the avocado, bananas, and coconut milk and blend well. Then, slowly add in the cacao, cinnamon, and monk fruit or stevia. Pour the mousse into a bowl and chill it in the fridge for one hour and then enjoy!

This recipe makes four servings.

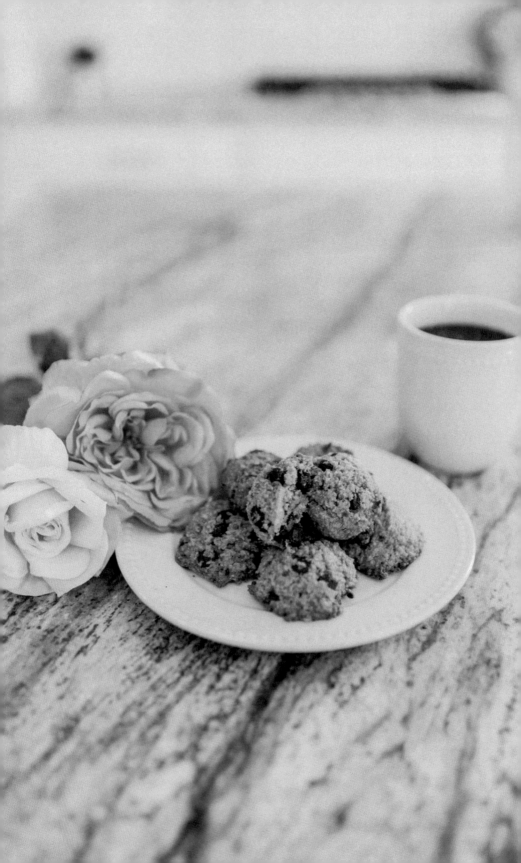

Coconut-Chocolate Chip Cookies

Almonds, coconut, and chocolate, oh my! This cookie is the perfect combination of these three delicious flavors! They are full of protein, fiber, and healthy fat as well! They really are the most amazing, chewy treat or snack any time of the day. Pair a couple with a cup of coffee and you will for sure be in love! Try them out! I know you will love them!

Ingredients

- 1 cup almond flour
- 1 cup shredded unsweetened coconut
- 3 eggs
- 1 tsp vanilla extract
- 1/2 cup coconut sugar
- 1/4 tsp salt
- 1/3 cup melted coconut oil
- 1/2 tsp baking powder
- 1/2 cup Enjoy Life chocolate chips

Directions

Preheat your oven to 350°F. Then, in a medium bowl, combine the above ingredients, leaving the chocolate chips for last. Then, slowly fold in the chocolate chips. Lastly, with a two-inch cookie or ice-cream scoop, portion out the cookie dough onto a greased baking sheet or Pyrex dish. Bake the cookies for 15-20 minutes or until slightly golden brown.

*This recipe makes about twelve cookies.

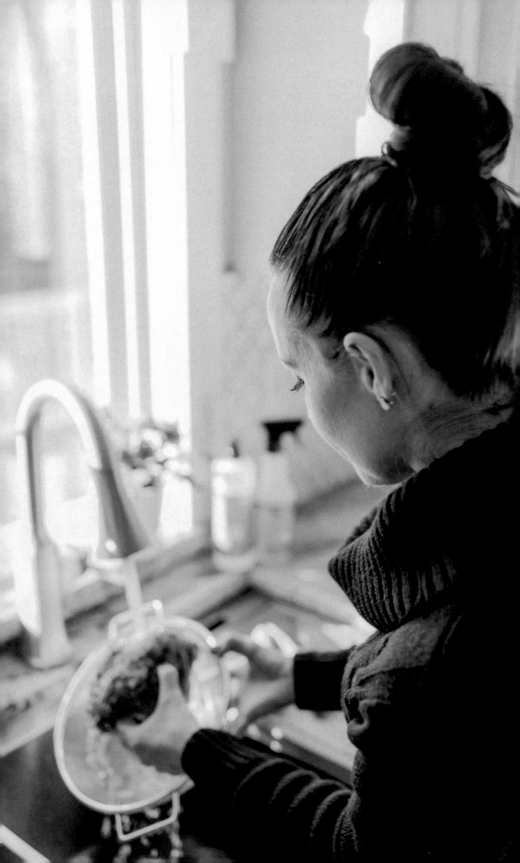

Live Healthy with Laura's 5-Day Meal Plan & Grocery List

The best way to gain confidence in the kitchen is simply to get in there and give it a go! The more time you spend in the kitchen, the more confident and adventurous you will become! Devote a couple of hours this weekend to grocery shop for these items and prep for the week ahead! Now, listen, I totally get it. We all can feel that there is just no time left to meal prep in our busy lives. But if we want to really better our health, we have to make and take the time. I have listed which recipes I suggest you prepare this weekend to ensure next week will go more smoothly for you! Please don't let this "meal prep" list intimidate you. You will be amazed at how simple my recipes are to make and at how much easier your week will be after taking the time to plan and think ahead! You also will be eating delicious food all week long and nourishing your body with the micro- and macronutrients it needs at the same time! You really can't go wrong! Now, let's get to baking and cooking recipes straight from my kitchen, and let's bring them to yours!

Weekend Prep

- Almond Butter Fruit Dip (prep time: 5 minutes)
- Feta, Tomato & Quinoa Salad (prep time: 10 minutes)
- Honey & Cinnamon-Roasted Chickpeas (prep time: 5 minutes)
- Strawberry No-Bake Energy Bars (prep time: 15 minutes)
- Cranberry & Walnut Tuna Salad (prep time: 10 minutes)
- Kale Chips (prep time: 5 minutes)
- Crunchy Peanut Butter Cookies (prep time: 15 minutes)
- Cinnamon-Raisin Muffins (prep time: 15 minutes)
- Avocado-Chocolate Mousse (prep time: 5 minutes)

Total Prep Time: 1 hour and 25 minutes (not including baking time)

5-Day Meal Plan

Monday (Day One)

Breakfast	Blueberry & Avocado Smoothie (make the morning of in 5 minutes)
Snack	Almond Butter Fruit Dip & Apple Slices
Lunch	Feta, Tomato & Quinoa Salad
Snack	Honey & Cinnamon-Roasted Chickpeas
Dinner	Baked Turkey Meatballs over Zucchini Pasta in Garlic Butter (prep time: 20 minutes)
Dessert	Avocado-Chocolate Mousse

Tuesday (Day Two)

Breakfast	Spinach & Feta Burrito (freeze the remaining burritos for later)
Snack	Strawberry No-Bake Energy Bars
Lunch	Cranberry & Walnut Tuna Salad
Snack	Kale Chips
Dinner	Broccoli & Salmon Curry Stir-fry (prep time: 15 minutes)
Dessert	Crunchy Peanut Butter Cookies

Wednesday (Day Three)

Breakfast	Cinnamon-Raisin Muffins
Snack	Almond Butter Fruit Dip & Apple Slices
Lunch	Feta, Tomato & Quinoa Salad
Snack	Honey & Cinnamon-Roasted Chickpeas
Dinner	Honey-BBQ Chicken Tenderloins with Steamed Broccoli (prep time: 15 minutes)
Dessert	Avocado-Chocolate Mousse and prep Overnight Chia Seed Pudding (prep time: 5 minutes)

Thursday (Day Four)

Breakfast	*Overnight Chia Seed Pudding*
Snack	*Strawberry No-Bake Energy Bars*
Lunch	*Cranberry & Walnut Tuna Salad*
Snack	*Kale Chips*
Dinner	*Goat Cheese & Sun-dried Tomato Rotini (prep time: 15 minutes)*
Dessert	*Crunchy Peanut Butter Cookies*

Friday (Day Five)

Breakfast	*Cinnamon-Raisin Muffins*
Snack	*Almond Butter Fruit Dip & Apple Slices*
Lunch	*Feta, Tomato & Quinoa Salad*
Snack	*Honey & Cinnamon-Roasted Chickpeas*
Dinner & Dessert	*"20 Night" (Relax, let go, and enjoy an entree, beverage, and dessert of YOUR choice!)*

Note: I created these dinner recipes with busy schedules in mind! On average, each dinner recipe in this meal plan should take you no more than 15-20 minutes to prepare, and they are designed to feed a *family of four*! Simply adjust the ingredients according to the size of your family or crowd!

Grocery List

This grocery list is the <u>exact list</u> of every item or product you will need in order to follow my meal plan this week! I recommend freezing any leftovers you may have for later!

Fruits

- 3/4 cup fresh blueberries
- 3 apples
- 3 ripe bananas
- 1 cup fresh strawberries
- 2/3 cups dried cranberries
- 1/2 cup raisins
- 4 oz fresh berries of choice

Vegetables

- 1 cup cherry tomatoes (halved)
- 4 large zucchini (or 8 cups "zoodles")
- 6 garlic cloves
- 8 cups baby spinach leaves
- 8 cups field greens
- 6 sticks celery
- 4 cups kale
- 8 cups fresh or frozen broccoli
- 1 1/3 cup unseasoned, sun-dried tomatoes

Protein Sources

- 1 jar natural almond butter
- 1 jar natural peanut butter
- 1/2 cup chopped almonds
- 1/2 cup chopped peanuts
- 25 oz canned chickpeas
- 1 lb ground turkey
- 16 oz or four small fillets wild Alaskan salmon

- 2 lbs boneless, skinless chicken tenderloins
- 4 packets or cans of tuna (in water)
- 9 eggs
- 1/4 cup flax seeds
- 1/2 cup chia seeds

Dairy & Dairy Alternatives

- 8 oz crumbled feta cheese
- 4 oz grated parmesan cheese
- 8 oz crumbled goat cheese
- 1/2 cup unsweetened coconut milk yogurt
- 1 cup unsweetened coconut milk
- 8 tbsp real butter

Gluten-Free Grains & Products

- 1 1/2 cups dry brown rice
- 1 cup dried quinoa
- 4 gluten-free tortillas
- 2 cups quick oats
- 2 cups almond flour
- 1/2 cup rice flour
- 16 oz gluten-free rotini

Healthy Fats

- 4 medium-large, ripe avocados
- Extra virgin olive oil (EVOO)
- Coconut oil (unrefined)
- Coconut shavings
- Real mayonnaise

Baking Goods & Herbs

- Raw honey
- Ground cinnamon
- Vanilla extract

- Ground black pepper
- Pink Himalayan salt
- Coconut sugar
- Italian seasoning
- Garlic powder
- 4 fresh, minced garlic cloves (not from a jar)
- Dried rosemary
- Dried basil
- Cacao powder
- Liquid monk fruit or stevia
- Curry powder
- Nutritional yeast
- Baking powder (aluminum-free)
- Pure maple syrup
- Apple cider vinegar (with the "mother")
- Ketchup (high-fructose corn-syrup-free)
- Paprika
- Worcestershire sauce

Note: Keep in mind that when you are investing in baking and cooking supplies and seasonings, once you buy them, they will last you for many recipes to come in the future! Oftentimes, I only need to purchase some of these listed twice a year! Remember, a little goes a long way!

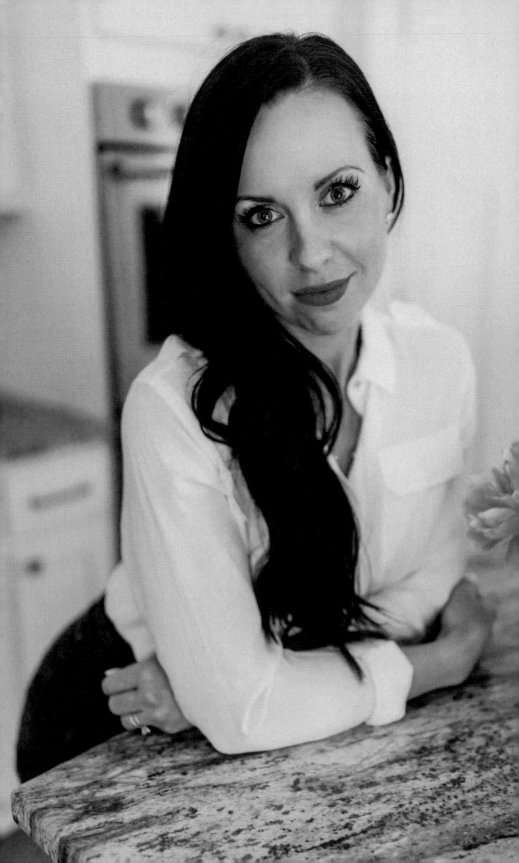

One Last Word Before You Go

Close your eyes for a moment. Picture yourself one year from now. How do you want to feel? What do you want to achieve by then? What do you want to find freedom from? Whatever your answers may be, I want you to remember that nothing with God is out of our reach. We should always strive to feel and be our best, and we should <u>always</u> dream big. When we do, we are able to enjoy this beautiful life far more, take risks, and find success, and we are able to offer ourselves more fully to those we love. "Settling" is just not part of our story! You and I were made for greatness, and we have SO much to achieve!

However, in order to achieve what we were meant to on this earth, we <u>must</u> care for our bodies both mentally and physically. They are the vessels that take us through our lives. When we fuel them well and treat them with love and respect, they will have the stamina to help us achieve our goals and unique purposes here on this earth. Our health should not be viewed as an uphill battle but instead as a journey. Our journey may have hills, bumps, and valleys, but nevertheless, it keeps going. It really is a beautiful, rewarding journey. Forget the scale for a moment and ask yourself every day: How do I feel? What is my body needing from me to function at its prime and feel its best?

When we stop viewing self-care as negotiable, and we take the time to fuel, move, and rest our body properly, we are truly able to thrive! Reaching our healthiest weight and best physique is a natural side effect to a healthy, balanced life.

So, get in that kitchen, my friend, and discover what foods make you feel vibrant, satisfied, and energized. Burn those muffins, drop some eggshells in that batter, and then laugh it off and start over. Trust me, it's all part of the process, and it's totally okay! Give yourself grace. Try out new exercises until you find one that suits you, and don't think twice about what is "trending." Practice saying "no" and allow your body time to rest and recover when it is telling you it needs a break. Live a little and let go of the things that aren't worth stressing over and which are out of your control. Indulge in moderation in the foods that you love, and don't give yourself any grief about it. Take a chance and be willing to make mistakes. Laugh a lot and surround yourself with those who make you feel uplifted, supported, loved, and appreciated. Count your blessings every day, and lastly, never forget that YOU are worth it!

With love,
Laura

Made in the USA
Middletown, DE
23 January 2021